Selected Topics in Prenatal and Neonatal Diagnoses

Edited by Irina Vlasova-St. Louis

Published in London, United Kingdom

Selected Topics in Prenatal and Neonatal Diagnoses
http://dx.doi.org/10.5772/10.5772/intechopen.111037
Edited by Irina Vlasova-St. Louis

Contributors
Alexandra Matei, Irina Vlasova-St. Louis, Madhavi Latha Routhu, Svetlana Khaiboullina, Thalía Harmony, Uri Barak

First published in London, United Kingdom, 2025 by IntechOpen
IntechOpen is the global imprint of INTECHOPEN LIMITED, registered in England and Wales, registration number: 11086078, 167-169 Great Portland Street, London, W1W 5PF, United Kingdom

For EU product safety concerns: IN TECH d.o.o., Prolaz Marije Krucifikse Kozulić 3, 51000 Rijeka, Croatia, info@intechopen.com or visit our website at intechopen.com.

British Library Cataloguing-in-Publication Data
A catalogue record for this book is available from the British Library

Selected Topics in Prenatal and Neonatal Diagnoses
Edited by Irina Vlasova-St. Louis
p. cm.

This title is part of the Obstetrics and Gynecology Book Series, Volume 6
Topic: Maternal-fetal Medicine
Series Editor: Zouhair O. Amarin
Topic Editor: Artúr Beke

Print ISBN 978-0-85466-878-6
Online ISBN 978-0-85466-877-9
eBook (PDF) ISBN 978-0-85466-879-3
ISSN 3049-706X

IntechOpen Book Series
Obstetrics and Gynecology
Volume 6

Aims and Scope of the Series

Obstetrics and Gynecology field typically covers several subspecialties that include maternal-fetal medicine, gynecologic oncology, reproductive endocrinology and subfertility, urogynecology and female pelvic reconstructive surgery, critical care medicine, complex family planning, pediatric and adolescent gynecology, menopausal and geriatric gynecology, and minimally invasive gynecologic surgery.
Apart from being diverse, obstetrics and gynecology is a challenging and demanding specialty. It combines medical and surgical skills.
The sequence of books in this series will have certain characteristics in common that will be recognized as part of the same informative multi-volume book programme.

Meet the Series Editor

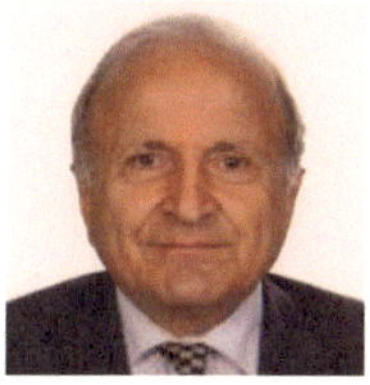

Zouhair Amarin is a Professor of Obstetrics and Gynaecology at the Jordan University of Science and Technology. He was previously a lecturer at the University of Glasgow, Scotland, a senior lecturer at the University of Nottingham, England, and the dean of the Faculty of Medicine at Mutah University, Jordan. Professor Amarin is a fellow of the Royal College of Obstetricians and Gynaecologists, and the Faculty of Public Health, London. He holds master's degrees in medical science and medical education. He is a pioneer in IVF and was the first in the world to develop microsurgical epididymis sperm aspiration for clinical use. He also discovered a surgical procedure for critical ovarian hyperstimulation syndrome. Professor Amarin has edited books, authored book chapters, and published more than 130 papers. He is the recipient of eight awards.

Meet the Volume Editor

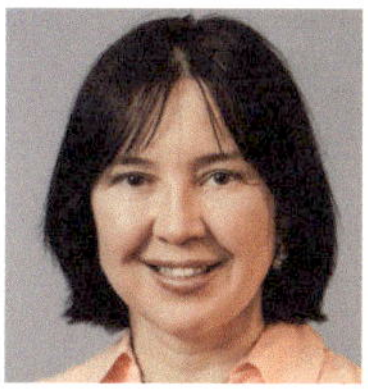

Dr. Vlasova-St. Louis is a distinguished biomedical specialist with extensive expertise in molecular medicine. She earned her MD and Ph.D. from Ural State Medical Academy in Russia, followed by postdoctoral training at the University of Minnesota in the USA and a fellowship sponsored by the Lymphoma Research Foundation. Utilizing cutting-edge techniques such as next-generation sequencing, she has made significant biomedical discoveries across molecular, cellular, and organismal levels in both normal and pathological conditions. As an Assistant Professor in the Division of Infectious Diseases and International Medicine at the University of Minnesota, Dr. Vlasova-St. Louis led research on immune reconstitution in immunocompromised individuals. She collaborated with the Division of Hematology-Oncology and Transplantation to study complications arising from various conditioning therapies and hematopoietic stem cell transplantation regimens. Additionally, she was a genomics specialist at the Newborn Molecular Analysis Unit, contributing to public health initiatives in newborn screening through advanced sequencing programs. Currently, Dr. Vlasova-St. Louis is the President of Vinnana AI LLC, an AI-driven company specializing in genetic variant interpretation. She has an extensive record of scientific publications in high-impact journals, books, and conference presentations, solidifying her reputation as a leader in molecular medicine and genomic research.

Contents

Preface

The future of perinatal care lies in precision medicine,
early intervention, and a commitment to giving
every newborn the healthiest start in life.
— Adapted from modern medical perspectives —

The rapid evolution of medical science continues to transform our understanding of prenatal and neonatal health. With technological advancements and deeper insights into fetal and neonatal physiology, clinicians and researchers are better equipped than ever to diagnose and manage conditions that impact the earliest stages of life. *Selected Topics in Prenatal and Neonatal Diagnoses* brings together a curated selection of contemporary research and clinical advancements highlighting the significant strides made in early detection and intervention.

The introductory chapter, *Advances in Prenatal and Neonatal Diagnostics*, provides a comprehensive overview of recent progress in this field, setting the stage for the specialized topics that follow. Among these is the application of ultrasound volumetric imaging in detecting fetal central nervous system anomalies. This technique enhances diagnostic accuracy, allowing for earlier and more precise assessments of fetal brain development. Another chapter delves into the role of ultrasound and its recent applications in diagnosing fetal malformations, underscoring its significance as a non-invasive, accessible, and indispensable tool in prenatal care.

Genetic advancements have revolutionized diagnostic capabilities. Next-generation sequencing (NGS) and variant cataloging are now essential tools for screening and diagnosing lysosomal storage disorders, including sphingolipidoses and mucopolysaccharidoses. This volume explores how these advanced methodologies enhance genetic diagnostics, refine risk assessments, and deepen our understanding of disease pathogenesis and progression in affected neonates.

Beyond diagnostics, early interventions are pivotal in shaping neonatal outcomes. One chapter of this book examines Katona's neurorehabilitation procedure, which harnesses neuroplasticity to support recovery. This approach introduces targeted rehabilitation techniques designed to mitigate long-term impairments, offering hope for infants affected by perinatal brain injuries.

This volume aims to serve as a valuable resource for clinicians and medical professionals dedicated to maternal-fetal and neonatal health. By bridging the gap between innovative research and clinical practice, we hope to contribute to the ongoing efforts to improve diagnostic precision and therapeutic outcomes for the most vulnerable patients - those at the very beginning of life.

We extend our deepest gratitude to the contributing authors for their dedication and expertise and to the readers seeking to expand their knowledge in this ever-evolving field. May this book inspire further inquiry and innovation in prenatal and neonatal medicine.

Irina Vlasova-St. Louis
The President of Vinnana AI LLC,
Jackson, USA

Chapter 1

Introductory Chapter: Advances in Prenatal and Neonatal Diagnostics

Irina Vlasova-St. Louis

1. Introduction

Maternal and fetal health are fundamental predictors of an individual's well-being throughout life, extending from infancy through childhood, adolescence, and adulthood. Early diagnosis and management of prenatal and neonatal diseases are crucial to ensuring optimal outcomes for newborns and reducing the long-term burden of neurodevelopmental impairments and physical disabilities. In this context, the emergence of advanced technologies has led to the integration of ultrasound imaging, mass spectrometry, genetic sequencing, and wearable devices into clinical practice (**Figure 1**).

2. Modern diagnostics

Over the past few decades, advancements in ultrasound technology have significantly improved. Ultrasound is now routinely used during the first trimester of pregnancy for early screening and diagnosis. Ultrasound can confirm the viability

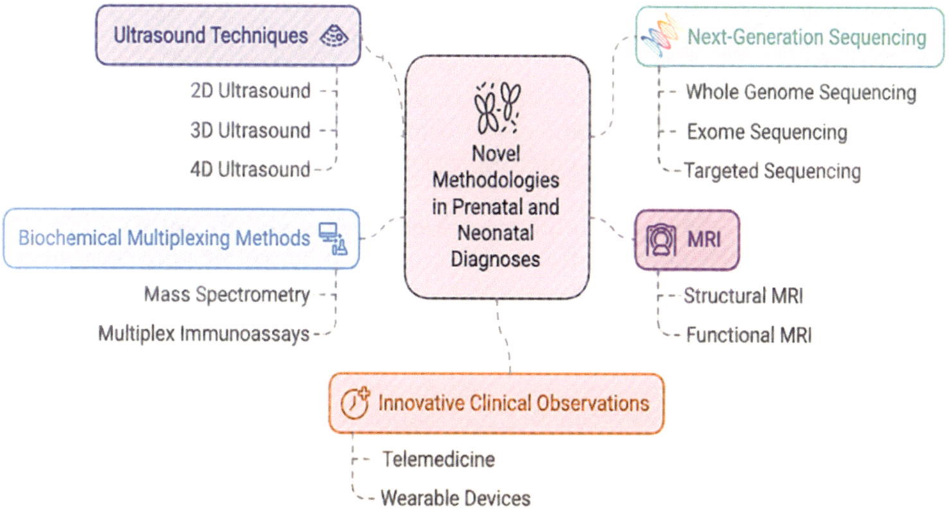

Figure 1.
Applications of novel diagnostics in prenatal and neonatal medicine.

of pregnancy, assess gestational age, and detect multiple pregnancies or structural anomalies, such as neural tube or abdominal wall defects.

High fetal imaging quality can now be obtained during first-trimester of pregnancy, providing clearer, more detailed images and enabling earlier detection of congenital abnormalities (e.g., evaluation of nuchal translucency) and monitoring fetal development (more description is provided in this book) [1]. The replacement of high-frequency 2-dimentional ultrasound with 3D and 4D HD imaging techniques (**Figure 1**) has improved the accuracy of diagnosing internal organ anomalies, facial anomalies, and other skeletal malformations, which accompany various chromosomal and congenital diseases [2]. They also add the dimension of real-time motion, assessing fetal movements and behaviors, such as facial expressions, which can provide insights into neurological development [1]. Doppler ultrasound measures placental and fetal/placental/umbilical cord blood circulation, detecting conditions such as intrauterine growth restriction and fetal hypoxia [3]. Transfontanelle ultrasound is commonly used in neonates, particularly premature infants, to assess the brain for abnormalities [4]. In some cases, ultrasound can be followed up by MRI, to improve resolution of brain and other tissues [5]. Advancements in instrument portability, along with the integration of tablets connected to cloud-based interfaces, have streamlined diagnostic protocols and significantly accelerated the interpretation of imaging results [6, 7]. Artificial intelligence (AI) and machine learning algorithms can assist in identification of subtle anomalies prenatally and in neonates, improving diagnostic accuracy and reducing operator dependency [6].

High-throughput biochemical technologies like liquid chromatography tandem mass spectrometry (LC-MS/MS) offer tests that can multiplex the detection of several biochemical biomarkers [8]. These tests become invaluable as a dry blood spot-based newborn screening tests for inborn error of metabolism disorders [8]. Early detection of metabolic disorders through mass spectrometry-based newborn screening allows for the initiation of life-saving treatments. These may include dietary modifications, enzyme replacement therapies, and, in severe cases, hematopoietic stem cell transplantation [9, 10]. With support from machine learning infrastructure, metabolomic diagnostics hold promise for improving newborn health by enabling early detection of metabolic disorders, which could ultimately reduce the long-term economic burden of disease treatment and management if integrated into routine care [11].

Genetic tests become integral to diagnosing rare genetic disorders, where standard diagnostic tools fall short. Noninvasive prenatal testing (NIPT) is a tool for screening pregnant women for fetal chromosomal aneuploidies [12]. NIPT detects cell-free fetal DNA (cffDNA) circulating in the maternal bloodstream as early as 9 weeks of gestation [12, 13]. Next-generation cffDNA sequencing (NGS-NIPT) is routinely used for detecting chromosomal aneuploidies, significantly reducing the need for invasive procedures such as amniocentesis or chorionic villus sampling for confirmatory testing [13]. Recent advancements in NIPT technologies have enabled screening for pathogenic microdeletions, fetal RhD status, and fetal sex determination where there is a risk of X-linked genetic disorders. Although NIPT is highly accurate for detecting common trisomies, its accuracy decreases for macrodeletions and sex chromosome abnormalities [14]. Research is underway to develop NIPT technologies capable of whole-genome sequencing (WGS), which would allow for the screening of a broader range of genetic conditions and could potentially include monogenic disorders, rare genetic syndromes, and screening for multiple pregnancies [15, 16].

NGS-based genomics newborn screening (GNS) has become an invaluable tool in neonatal care units, offering life-saving diagnostic capabilities for newborns with rare genetic conditions, enabling neonatologists and pediatricians to intervene promptly, tailoring treatment strategies to the individual needs of the newborn [17]. The GNS program provides significant benefits in improving neonatal health outcomes and ending diagnostic odyssey early [18]. There have been proposals of expansion on GNS as the first-tier screening, which would precede traditional biochemical methods [19]. Yet many challenges remain in the interpretation of genetic test results, such as reporting variants of uncertain significance (VUS), which may lead to referral for additional testing, and anxiety for parents about child's future health [20, 21]. NGS-based carrier screening of recessive diseases and genetic counseling of carrier-parents, who are at risk of having offspring with known pathogenic gene variants, gives the option to make informed decisions about current or future pregnancies [22].

Thorough clinical assessment is still essential part of early diagnostics of newborns and should not be disregarded. Perinatal brain damage, resulting from complications such as hypoxic-ischemic encephalopathy, intracranial hemorrhage, or preterm births, often results in motor, cognitive, and developmental challenges, including cerebral palsy, epilepsy, and intellectual disabilities [23, 24]. By leveraging the brain's natural plasticity, targeted rehabilitation techniques, like Katona's method, described in this book, was designed to mitigate long-term neurological consequences. Katona's approach leverages newborn's neuroplasticity, using structured repetition of reflexes to form new neural pathways that compensate for brain damage [25]. Additionally, the integration of wearable devices and telemedicine into neonatal care enhances early detection and continuous monitoring, allowing for real-time assessment of vital signs, movement patterns, and neurological function (**Figure 1**). These technologies facilitate timely interventions, particularly in remote or underserved areas, improving long-term outcomes.

3. Conclusion

The field of prenatal and neonatal diagnostics has seen remarkable advancements. The combination of molecular and biochemical diagnostics with advance imaging holds great promise for improving the health newborns through implementation of preventive measures and individualized treatments. Moreover, genome editing technologies are now applied as targeted treatments of malfunctioning genes, offering opportunities to treat fetus during pregnancy [26]. The ultimate goal is to deliver timely preventive measures and ensure each person receives the most appropriate treatment when needed.

While novel diagnostics require significant expertise and infrastructure, their value in detecting and managing perinatal diseases is immeasurable. However, these advances bring challenges, particularly in terms of cost, accessibility, and the need for highly skilled personnel.

Author details

Irina Vlasova-St. Louis
Vinnana AI LLC, USA

*Address all correspondence to: stlouil@alumni.jh.edu

References

[1] Leung K. Applications of advanced ultrasound technology in obstetrics. Diagnostics (Basel). 2021;**11**(7):1-18

[2] Recker F, Gembruch U, Strizek B. Clinical ultrasound applications in obstetrics and gynecology in the year 2024. Journal of Clinical Medicine. 2024;**13**(5):1-6

[3] Chen JY, Yu BL, Wu XJ, Li YF, Zhong LY, Chen M. A longitudinal and cross-sectional study of placental circulation between normal and placental insufficiency pregnancies. Placenta (Eastbourne). 2024;**149**:29-36

[4] Hadžić D. Transfontaneal brain ultrasound: A powerful assessment tool for critically ill neonates. Research in Education and Rehabilitation. 2023;**6**(1):108-117

[5] Cawley P, Padormo F, Cromb D, Almalbis J, Marenzana M, Teixeira R, et al. Development of neonatal-specific sequences for portable ultralow field magnetic resonance brain imaging: A prospective, single-centre, cohort study Research in context. EClinicalMedicine. 2023;**65**:102253

[6] Yee WLS, Drum CL. Increasing complexity to simplify clinical care: High resolution mass spectrometry as an enabler of ai guided clinical and therapeutic monitoring. Advanced Therapeutics. 2020;**3**(4):1-6

[7] Plöger R, Behning C, Walter A, Jimenez Cruz J, Gembruch U, Strizek B, et al. Next-generation monitoring in obstetrics: Assessing the accuracy of non-piezo portable ultrasound technology. Acta Obstetricia et Gynecologica Scandinavica. 2024;**103**(10):2031-2041

[8] Gelb MH, Basheeruddin K, Burlina A, Chen H, Chien Y, Dizikes G, et al. Liquid chromatography-tandem mass spectrometry in newborn screening laboratories. International Journal of Neonatal Screening. 2022;**8**(4):62

[9] Millington DS. How mass spectrometry revolutionized newborn screening. Journal of Mass Spectrometry and Advances in the Clinical Lab. 2024;**32**:1-10

[10] Tan EY, Boelens JJ, Jones SA, Wynn RF. Hematopoietic stem cell transplantation in inborn errors of metabolism. Frontiers in Pediatrics. 2019;**7**:433

[11] Yang X, Ding S, Zhang J, Hu Z, Zhuang D, Wang F, et al. The significance of machine learning in neonatal screening for inherited metabolic diseases. Frontiers in Pediatrics. 2024;**12**:1366891

[12] Kwon H, Yun S, Joo J, Park D, Do W, Lee S, et al. Improving the accuracy of noninvasive prenatal testing through size-selection between fetal and maternal cfDNA. Prenatal Diagnosis. 2023;**43**(13):1581-1592

[13] Kwan AHW, Gil MM, Xue S, Kwok YKY, Lau D, Fung J, et al. Cell-free DNA test for fetal chromosomal abnormalities in multiple pregnancies. Acta Obstetricia et Gynecologica Scandinavica. 2024;**103**(9):1799-1807

[14] Eltabbakh N, Mohasin Y, Jeddy R. Advancements of non-invasive prenatal testing: the role of obstetricians. Frontiers in Medicine. 2024;**11**:1388481

[15] Audibert F, Wou K, Okun N, De Bie I, Wilson RD. Guideline No. 456:

Prenatal screening for fetal chromosomal anomalies. Journal of Obstetrics and Gynaecology Canada [Netherlands: Elsevier Inc]. 2024:102694, 1-10

[16] Qiao L. cfDNA from maternal plasma for noninvasive screening of fetal exomes. American Journal of Clinical and Experimental Immunology. 2024;**13**(1):56-57

[17] Jiang S, Wang H, Gu Y. Genome sequencing for newborn screening—An effective approach for tackling rare diseases. JAMA Network Open. 2023;**6**(9):e2331141

[18] Chen T, Fan C, Huang Y, Feng J, Zhang Y, Miao J, et al. Genomic sequencing as a first-tier screening test and outcomes of newborn screening. JAMA Network Open. 2023;**6**(9):e2331162

[19] Narravula A, Garber KB, Askree SH, Hegde M, Hall PL. Variants of uncertain significance in newborn screening disorders: Implications for large-scale genomic sequencing. Genetics in Medicine. 2017;**19**(1):77-82

[20] Kiewiet G, Westra D, De Boer EN, van Berkel E, Hofste TGJ, van Zweeden M, et al. Future of Dutch NGS-based newborn screening: Exploring the technical possibilities and assessment of a variant classification strategy. International Journal of Neonatal Screening. 2024;**10**(1):1-20

[21] Zhang X, Chen Q, Li J, Luo X, Luo J, Li J, et al. The effectiveness of expanded carrier screening based on next-generation sequencing for severe monogenic genetic diseases. Human Genomics. 2024;**18**(1):9-8

[22] Hyun SE, Kwon J, Hong BY, Yoon JA, Choi JY, Hong J, et al. Early neurodevelopmental assessments of neonates discharged from the neonatal intensive care unit: A physiatrist's perspective. Annals of Rehabilitation Medicine. 2023;**47**(3):147-161

[23] Hadders-Algra M. Early diagnostics and early intervention in neurodevelopmental disorders-age-dependent challenges and opportunities. Journal of Clinical Medicine. 2021;**10**(4):861

[24] Gonzalez-Moreira E, Harmony T, Hinojosa-Rodríguez M, Carrillo-Prado C, Juárez-Colín ME, Gutiérrez-Hernández CC, et al. Prevention of neurological sequelae in preterm infants. Brain Sciences. 2023;**13**(5):753

[25] Krbec BA, Zhang X, Chityat I, Brady-Mine A, Linton E, Copeland D, et al. Emerging innovations in neonatal monitoring: A comprehensive review of progress and potential for non-contact technologies. Frontiers in Pediatrics. 2024;**12**:1442753

[26] Mattar CNZ, Chan JKY, Choolani M. Gene modification therapies for hereditary diseases in the fetus. Prenatal Diagnosis. 2023;**43**(5):674-686

Chapter 2

Applicability of Ultrasound Volumetric Approach in the Prenatal Detection of Fetal CNS Anomalies

Alexandra Matei

Abstract

Accessibility to newer imaging technologies has led, over the last years, to improved detection of prenatal CNS anomalies. Considering the implications regarding poor prognosis and postnatal adverse fetal outcomes, the early detection rate is still considered unsatisfactory, mostly related to 2D ultrasound examinations, which are highly operator-dependent. Transvaginal 3D volumetric ultrasound offers the possibility of multiplanar analysis of fetal CNS architecture but requires a spatial sense of anatomic landmark distribution. Automated and semiautomated volumetric approaches are currently being studied, and promising results underline their advantages compared to fetal magnetic resonance imaging, which is time- and resource-consuming. 3D volume contrast imaging C (VCI-C) depicts considerable aspects of cerebellar and vermis morphology, allowing concomitant biometric measurements. The possibility to examine additional diagnostic planes increases vizualization of specific intracranial structures, leading to extensive insight into specific anomalies. Implementation of standard neurosonographic plane acquisition could overcome several downfalls of the ultrasound volumetric reconstruction approach.

Keywords: neurosonography, 3D ultrasound, fetal anomalies, multiplanar, volumetric, central nervous system

1. Introduction

Prenatal screening for fetal anomalies is routinely performed in obstetrical practice to detect life-threatening conditions. The development of *in-vivo* fetal imaging techniques, such as ultrasound and magnetic resonance imaging (MRI), marked a cornerstone in prenatal detection and assessment of central nervous system (CNS) malformations, an essential aspect of paramount importance in fetal wellbeing.

There is a reported high incidence of CNS malformations in as many as 1–2/1.000 fetuses, consequently accounting for the most common congenital abnormalities [1–3]. Neural tube defects are the most frequent CNS malformations, with a

 IntechOpen

prevalence in pregnancy of 52/100.000, but evidence suggests that cerebral structural anomalies with an intact neural tube might reach an incidence of approximately 1/100 births [3].

Basic mid-trimester transabdominal ultrasound examination of the fetal brain requires the acquisition of three views based on two axial planes: transventricular and transthalamic views required for the evaluation of brain hemispheres and an additional axial transcerebellar view necessary for the evaluation of the posterior fossa [4]. The following structures should be analyzed: cavum septum pellucidi, midline falx, thalami, lateral ventricles with choroid plexus, cerebellum and cisterna magna [4]. Whenever a fetal brain anomaly is suspected or the pregnancy is associated with high-risk for the development of the aforementioned conditions, experts rely on extended ultrasound examination. This comprehensive targeted evaluation is entitled "neurosonography". It is an advanced ultrasound assessment of the fetal CNS that implies up-to-date knowledge of fetal neurology and brain anatomy. Specific indications for targeted fetal neurosonography can be reviewed in the updated International Society of Ultrasound in Obstetrics and Gynecology (ISUOG) guideline dedicated to fetal CNS examination [2].

As mentioned before, suspicion of fetal CNS abnormalities leads to the necessity for further paraclinical investigations to disentangle doubtful diagnoses. In addition to mid-trimester transabdominal ultrasound, fetal neurosonography encompasses the transvaginal multiplanar approach and fetal MRI. Both ultrasound techniques offer the possibility to study brain growth and development during the fetal period using the volumetric approach. Fetal MRI is a non-invasive diagnostic tool that can characterize the development of the CNS due to increased image resolution and tissue contrast and therefore contributes to pregnancy management [5].

The basis for targeted ultrasound examination of fetal CNS is the multiplanar approach [3]. Compared to routine screening evaluation which focuses on three axial views obtained by transabdominal evaluation, neurosonography prioritizes the transvaginal examination when the fetus is in vertex presentation, due to the higher resolution of images allowing for appropriate display of additional coronal and sagittal planes. For other fetal presentations, an external version might be considered [3]. Four coronal views (transfrontal, transcaudate, transthalamic and transcerebellar) and three sagittal views (mid-sagittal anterior, mid-sagittal posterior, parasagittal) are recommended key planes, but additional views can be necessary for diagnosis, depending on the region of interest; combined approaches – transabdominal and transvaginal are sometimes required as well [3, 6].

In this context, the role of three-dimensional (3D) ultrasound is unquestionable, since it allows the operator to display and analyze simultaneously perfectly aligned views in all orthogonal planes, which also benefit from enhanced image quality [3]. Several international guidelines and protocols provide detailed instructions on the specific methodology required for the relevant acquisition of these views [2–4].

Depending on the resources each department benefits from, various imaging options have been proposed and studied in order to maximize the cost-benefit balance in the practice of prenatal fetal anomaly screening and diagnosis.

Conventional two-dimensional (2D) ultrasound is a powerful, real-time non-invasive and non-ionizing diagnostic tool in the hands of an experienced operator [7, 8]. It has broad clinical applicability, and the fact that it is a safe imaging technique, allows it to be the preferred diagnostic approach in fetal imaging.

In everyday obstetrical activity access to an ultrasound machine has become indispensable. Depending on the aim of the obstetrical evaluation, 2D ultrasound mode is an adequate resource for the assessment of fetal wellbeing and growth as well as for standard screening for structural anomalies. However, over the last couple of years, an increased requirement for additional ultrasound tools has emerged, especially to improve the detection rates during the performance of targeted sonography. This is mainly related to the operator-dependent imaging acquisition mode, which precisely influences the interpretation of ultrasound images and data. This is a consistent issue especially if the processes of acquisition and interpretation of images are performed by different people: a sonographer and/or a clinician/obstetrician, depending on the specific national health care system requirements.

Multiple clinical applications of 2D planar ultrasound imaging are relevant to the day-to-day obstetrical workflow. Several criteria have promoted this imaging system as a clinically accepted screening and diagnostic tool, mainly during prenatal follow-up: a fast, safe, economical and portable ultrasound examination usually provides a rapid and accurate assessment of both the fetus and the mother, reducing the length of stay in the clinic [9]. Compared to the MRI – the other medical imaging system available for use during pregnancy, which implies a significantly higher financial burden for any healthcare system as well as a time-consuming clinical activity, the 2D ultrasound evaluation offers an acceptably accurate examination in the hands of a skilled user, enough to justify its operation and maintenance costs [9]. The set of images provided and stored by MRI examination are undoubtedly superior but still sensitive to fetal motion artifacts.

On the other hand, the 2D scan allows the user to identify images of different sections of 3D fetal anatomical structures, but in the absence of an automatic frame of reference, the exact orientation of the image is not precisely determined since it is strongly dependent on the hand positioning of the ultrasound probe. Therefore, there is an increased variability in the image acquisition process, although in clinical practice obstetrical guidelines offer strong recommendations concerning the standard views to be used in fetal anomaly screening and diagnosis as well as the anatomical landmarks to aid measurements and localize probe position and orientation [9].

Volumetric 3D ultrasound aims to surpass the operator-dependent characteristic of standard 2D scans, by using specialized probes. By performing a volumetric 3D scan of different sections of the body using a standard, anatomically registered frame of reference, this examination offers the possibility to swipe through a set of individual images belonging to a block of dataset, allowing the user to access sagittal, transverse and/or coronal planes.

Potential limitations that encourage continuous research for more complex and advanced image acquisition strategies refer to the small field of view, limited penetration, diffraction-limited resolution and the fact that a 2D image yields only a selective cross-sectional sampling of a complete 3D anatomical volume; consequently, a significant level of skill and experience are essential for the user to obtain a recognizable, clinically useful, high-quality ultrasound image [7, 10].

Performing a fetal scan either for screening of fetal anomalies or for evaluation of fetal growth is routine practice during prenatal visits. As mentioned before, depending on the aim of the evaluation, capturing in detail a region of interest has become a necessity. Volumetric 3D ultrasound imaging has emerged as a solution for this, based on the motor-controller "wobbler probe" with the internal motorized translation of a one-dimensional array and 2D "matrix array probes", which allow for acoustic beam steering in the elevation dimension in addition to the azimuth dimension [7, 9]. Nevertheless, image processing and interpretation are still dependent on the operator's skills, requiring advanced knowledge and experience to obtain maximum information related to the region of interest.

Ultrasound probes using sensing technologies to achieve volumetric image reconstruction represent an alternative to volumetric 3D ultrasound and have been investigated since the beginning of the 1990s. The main difference between them and the classic 2D probe technology resides in the integration of real-time tracking of the position and orientation of the probe and its acquired image data in 3D space [9]. To achieve this, a reference frame meaning a 3D Cartesian coordinate system must be established, and the transformation between each object specified; spatial location tracking is a functional requirement and is obtained using an electromagnetic field sensor or pre-calibrated optical tracking setup to retund both spatial coordinates and quaternions – the accepted standard parameterization of rotation [7].

Researchers at Stanford and Duke University have addressed the increasing demand for financially accessible alternatives and have developed setup devices that do not involve the high costs of the 3D ultrasound equipment mentioned above, but further improvements are needed [7, 9]. Current studies are focused on increasing the accuracy and intuitiveness of ultrasound image acquisition, with less reliance on operator skills; this way, several emerging tracking technologies – although still in the research stage, have proved significant potential to overcome current difficulties regarding motion artifacts and imaging resolution [11, 12]. In the era of the artificial intelligence breakthrough, it has become increasingly necessary to reach high rates of reproducibility in the field of diagnostic imaging by promoting automatization as part of medical progress.

Furthermore, the fetal automatic segmentation is of particular interest at present, since this would represent a pragmatic solution to the abovementioned downfalls of both 2D and 3D volumetric ultrasound approaches. Particularly referred to the challenges associated with the volumetric ultrasound of the whole fetal head; automatic solutions are currently sought to overcome:

- the poor image quality resulting from the speckle noise and low resolution

- low tissue contrast and long-span shadow occlusion caused by the significant acoustic attenuation on the skull

- the large variety of fetal heads, mainly inner structures' morphology during different gestational periods and fetal poses [13]

Multiple attempts have been dedicated to meet these challenges and even to simultaneously segment the fetus, gestational sac and placenta in ultrasound volumes [14].

However, neuroimaging studies during the fetal period began to advance almost two decades ago. Brain structure segmentation is an important prerequisite for identifying and labelling brain regions and deriving more accurate quantitative measurements [5, 15]. These measurements of the fetal brain and subcortical volumes can facilitate the early identification of predictors for brain dysmaturation [1]. Early detection of fetal brain abnormalities is of key clinical importance due to its involvement in obstetrical management of the affected pregnancies and the potential prediction of neurodevelopmental outcomes.

Several studies have focused on the potential of artificial intelligence to automatically segment brain tissue compartments using MRI, to address the issue of manual segmentation, which requires time and expertise; results showed significant efficacy and reproducibility of the conceived mechanisms, especially for the segmentation of the cerebellum and thalami – key cerebral structures involved in neurocognition and motor behavior [1, 5, 15]. Still, compared to MRI imaging, fetal sonography is strictly dependent on tissue properties and the positioning of the area of interest relative to the ultrasound transducer: anatomical boundaries are typically incomplete, and strong acoustic shadowing can interfere with image acquisition [16]. Initial studies focused on automatic ultrasound detection of specific fetal brain structures but currently, there is growing interest in automatic segmentation techniques, which allow for additional depiction of the structure's shape and appearance [16]. Huang et al. studied two brain structures that have different ultrasound appearances: the choroid plexus and the corpus callosum and proposed a method that allowed for automatic biometry measurements with acceptable deviations compared to within human inter−/intraobserver deviations and a high region segmentation accuracy [16].

2. Fetal CNS examination in early gestation

Early detection of fetal structural abnormalities at 11 + 0 to 14 + 0 weeks of gestation is the primary objective of the first-trimester morphology scan. ISUOG recommends that this examination should not be limited only to the assessment of fetal crown-rump length (CRL) and nuchal translucency (NT) [17] but should also encomprise a throughout evaluation of fetal anatomy, suggesting that adequate time allocated for a detailed structural survey can increase the detection rate.

Nevertheless, several synergistic factors influence the possibility of ultrasound detection of fetal structural anomalies. The type and quality of ultrasound equipment available for routine screening is an essential element to be considered. This is even more relevant if taking into consideration second-opinion scans or targeted fetal sonographies. Additionally, in these particular cases, the experience and skills of the examiner play a significant role in reaching a successful, complete and correct examination. In the process of ultrasound screening for anomalies, the sonographer needs to consider the epidemiological aspects related to potential structural defects that can be identified in the specific population and at a specific time in pregnancy.

In the first trimester of pregnancy, the main advantage of ultrasound screening resides in the fact that transvaginal probes can be used for adequate image acquisition, allowing excellent representation of fetal brain structures. However, at this early stage in pregnancy, manipulation of the fetus for optimal depiction of morphology corresponding to specific anatomical structures is extremely limited. This is where the value of 3D ultrasound specifically emerges. Experts in the field suggest that the fetal brain can be accurately assessed as early as 7 weeks of pregnancy, stating that embryological development can be followed using ultrasound, allowing for holoprosencephaly, anencephaly and spina bifida to be discovered early in the first trimester [18, 19].

Development of the fetal brain is a dynamic process and ultrasound evaluation of cerebral structures should take into account the rapid changes that the fetal CNS undergoes from the early to the mid and second half of gestation. Advances in imaging technology have known a breakthrough over the past three decades, allowing for studies to address the issues of early detection of fetal CNS anomalies. Early fetal neurosonography at 12–15 weeks of gestation allows for a throughout visualization of brain structures using a high-frequency transvaginal transducer [2, 3, 20], especially since the ossification process of the calvarium is not complete.

At 13–14 weeks of gestation, the focus should be on appraising the normal structure of the diencephalon and the posterior fossa, taking into consideration the fact that complete development of the cerebellum takes place later, in the second trimester, and therefore, suspected isolated vermian abnormalities at this stage in pregnancy associate high-risk of false-positive results [3, 19]. In this latter situation, mid-sagittal views can distinguish between normal development of posterior fossa structures and potential structural anomalies. New studies and protocols address the potential of early spina bifida diagnosis; specifically, the mid-sagittal plane allows the examiner to identify indirect signs and to perform custom measurements depicting the ratio between the brain stem and the distance between the brain stem to the occipital bone which in open spina bifida is >1 [3, 21]. Furthermore, Ushakov underlined the importance of 3D ultrasound volume acquisition at the first-trimester scan when he described "the crash sign" detectable on axial views in fetuses with spina bifida, marking the posterior displacement of the mesencephalon and deformation against the occipital bone [22]. However, as Paladini and Volpe anticipated more than 10 years ago, open spina bifida, cystic major anomalies of the posterior fossa and cerebral ventriculomegaly should remain "potentially detectable abnormalities" during early scans in pregnancy [19].

Specialized literature and internationally up-to-date protocols and guidelines recommend that despite the increasing performance in early neurosonography, a follow-up scan at 20 weeks of gestation should be performed in all pregnancies [3, 19]. Only particular cases of holoprosencephaly, anencephaly and gross cephalocele should disregard this recommendation since these entities should be clear-cut pathological entities to be recognized during first-trimester scan [3, 19].

3. Fetal CNS examination in later gestation

Ultrasound screening for fetal anomalies has been a routine assessment at mid-gestation for more than four decades. Specifically related to the evaluation of the fetal CNS, axial planes have been used for ensuring biometrical measurements and anatomical depiction of the main visible cephalic structures.

While for low-risk populations this protocol for basic examination covers sufficiently the need for prenatal morphological assessment of the fetus, in high-risk populations when suspicion of abnormal development occurs, additional investigations are required. Initially, MRI offered a feasible alternative for the detailed characterization of specific regions of interest and the surrounding areas of the fetal brain, mainly due to its quality as a non-ionizing radiation exposure imaging technique. Nevertheless, associated increased costs and timing for image acquisition, combined with restricted accessibility, emphasized the requirement for ultrasound technologists to provide solutions that would overcome the abovementioned downfalls.

Early studies on retrieving 3D ultrasound volumes began 30 years ago when researchers focused on precise quantitative volume measurement of fetal organs [23]. Rapid evolution in the field started with the construction of reference centiles based on the assessment of fetal brain volume and led in over a decade to a persistent search for improved solutions for more complex clinical issues related to the practice of prenatal anomaly screening: for example, refining the diagnostic ultrasound accuracy for fetal craniofacial dysmorphisms using shape optimization processes after fetal head segmentation [23, 24]. In parallel, comprehensive studies were conducted to identify normal global growth trajectory of fetal cerebral structures such as the cortical plate, deep gray nuclei and ventricles, using MRI [25]. It is already known that brain maturation takes place in the latter half of the pregnancy and that its structure has specific features during cerebral expansion. Disruptions of the expansion processes affecting the growth and regression of certain brain structures are suspected to determine the cognitive outcome of the fetus [25]. Therefore, it is of paramount importance to recognize the contribution MRI and histopathological studies had to the understanding of brain development; improving the slice thickness as part of the advanced image processing techniques to adjust the inter-slice motion and obtain a super-resolution reconstruction of volumetric images maintained fetal brain volumetry examinations essential in the evaluation of fetal development [26].

However, by using only the transverse plane of the fetal head, limited information can be obtained; consequently, the need for further evaluation of the remaining orthogonal planes has become more valuable. This was in accordance with postnatal ultrasound examinations of the brain, carried out through the large fontanel, providing coronal and sagittal planes that did not serve neonatologists for comparison with prenatal images. It was in 2007 that ISUOG issued the first guideline addressing the need for extended CNS sonography, known as "fetal neurosonography" [2, 3]. This way, suspicious findings in the fetal brain would require additional coronal and sagittal planes as part of the extended ultrasound evaluation. As expected, depending on multiple maternal (increased body-mass index) and fetal factors (presentation, anterior placental insertion, multiple pregnancies, etc.), these additional cutting planes are sometimes difficult to obtain.

With the introduction of 3D and 4D ultrasound, volume data sets are generated, and these allow for any cutting planes to be subsequently reconstructed. In 2012, Chaoui et al. were among the first experts to present the clinical applications of multiplanar reconstruction using 3D sonography in fetal CNS evaluation [18]. The digital information stocked in one or multiple volumes can be examined either retrospectively by 3D scanning mode or live by 4D examination. The reconstruction of the plane of interest is performed after the acquisition of the volume, which is further displayed using volume rendering – a similar technique to the one used for MRI and CT scanning.

Different representations of the cutting plane are possible: as a single cutting plane, as three orthogonal planes or as tomography – multiple very thin layer planes using volume contrast mode imaging (VCI) as the default setting to minimize artifacts; additionally, the examiner can draw a line or a curve by himself which can serve as the basis for the creation of the image [18]. This virtual reconstruction of images facilitates access to structures that are not usually sonographically clearly visible during a standard transabdominal ultrasound, such as the corpus callosum and the cerebellar vermis – for these structures, if the fetus lies in cephalic presentation, a transvaginal scan is an alternative for assessing their morphology.

For volume recording, Chaoui recommends setting a cross-sectional plane of the fetal head, parallel to the skull base, containing the cavum septi pellucidi, using a sweep angle >50°, to cover the entire brain [18]. This way, multiplanar rendering offers the possibility to display the architecture of the falx cerebri with the cavum septi pellucidi, anterior and dorsal horns of the lateral ventricles, cortex, cerebellum and cisterna magna. Moreover, the Omniview application allows the sonographer to recreate both sagittal and coronal planes based on the same initial acquisition transverse plane, to further assess the structure of the corpus callosum, cerebellar vermis, anterior complex and longitudinal ventricular diameter (**Figure 1**) [18].

In specific, targeted cases, multiplanar rendering can be performed after recording a data volume based on a coronal plane, using the cavum as an anatomical

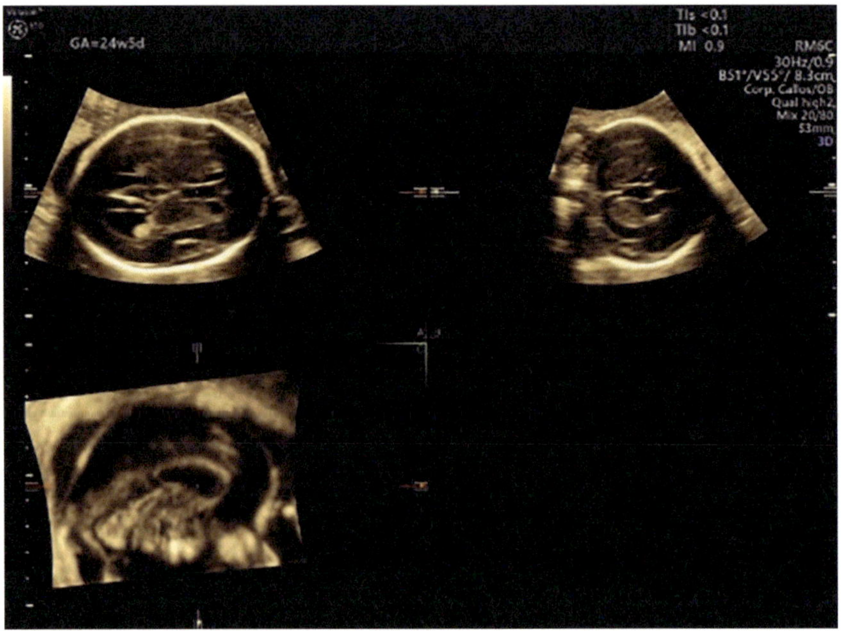

Figure 1.
Multiplanar examination of a fetal brain with suspected vermian hypoplasia at 24w5d scan. Based on transventricular view (plane A), coronal views (plane B) and sagittal views (plane C) allow for further analysis of corpus callosum or posterior fossa morphology. Personal archive.

landmark and a sweep angle >70° [18]. In this case, in addition to the previously mentioned structures, an image of the interhemispheric gap, the thalami, the lateral insulae as well as the gyri and sulci in the 3rd trimester can be analyzed [18]. In other words, suspected anomalies related to agenesis of the corpus callosum, to the anterior complex (anterior horn and cavum septi pellucidi) or the cortex, can be more precisely identified.

Gray matter migration process occurs in the 12th week of fetal development, which overlaps with the time of corpus callosum development; consequently, dysplasias of the corpus callosum can be accompanied by gray matter heterotopia [27]. Other CNS anomalies such as Dandy-Walker syndrome, absence of cavum septum pellucidi, Chiari malformation, septo-optic dysplasia, etc. can be identified concomitantly to corpus callosum dysplasia secondary to a neural tube disorder caused by specific adverse factors during the dorsal induction process of nerve end plate in the early embryonic development period [27].

A more detailed description of the corpus callosum morphology can be found in the reconstruction of the section based on the volume obtained using an initial sagittal plane of the fetal head and an acquisition angle >50°; in addition to the midline structures, the neighboring brain areas are also depicted and above all, an optimal display of genu, corpus, isthmus and splenium of the corpus callosum can be obtained, facilitating diagnosis of hypoplasia or other dysplasias of the corpus callosum [18]. Also, this is the preferred scan for cerebellar vermis assessment, including fissura prima, fissura secunda and brainstem to vermis angle [18], practical along with the transvaginal ultrasound, whenever anomalies of the fetal posterior fossa are suspected.

Reconstruction of the corpus callosum can be achieved after recording a volume data set based on a cross-sectional image of the fetal head, taking into account the following recommendations: to obtain the sagittal plane, the examiner must adjust the levels so that the A-axis lies in the same plane as the falx cerebri and the B plane perpendicular to the falx and the cavum septi pellucidi, thus resulting in a C-plane corresponding to the thalamus, cavum septi pellucidi and corpus callosum [18]. In a 4D scan, a line can be drawn by the sonographer directly on the region of interest.

Concomitantly, a similar reconstruction process can be performed to examine the cerebellar vermis further. If the basic ultrasound identifies suspicious findings in the area of the fetal posterior cranial fossa, additional sagittal exploration of the vermis and the surrounding structures needs to be accomplished. Reconstruction of this sagittal plane can be performed directly *via* the transcerebellar plane after volume acquisition, allowing the A-axis to pass through the vermis and the falx, and B plane perpendicular to the centre line; the C level will therefore visualize the vermis and the vermis-brain stem relation [18].

A more recent paper cites the applicability of the 3D volumetric transvaginal approach in the early characterization of posterior fossa structures, underlying the fact that the anterior membranous area and cerebellar vermis can be subject to in detail evaluation of their morphological changes even at first-trimester scan, as a basis for better understanding of pathological development of posterior fossa [28]. However, further research is needed before considering this approach in populational practice.

Experts mention that 3D ultrasound technologies such as volume contrast imaging in combination with C-plane (VCI-C) and tomographic ultrasound imaging (TUI) although used for the assessment of corpus callosum and vermis cerebelli, still have some limitations since they cannot clearly distinguish the corpus callosum from septum pellucidi because the acoustic beam is parallel to fetal head [27]. This is where the implementation of the 3D Omniview technique can provide the corresponding image of the region of interest by manually cutting using either a straight line (**Figures 2** and **3**) or a curvilinear approach to the 3D data in an arbitrary direction [27].

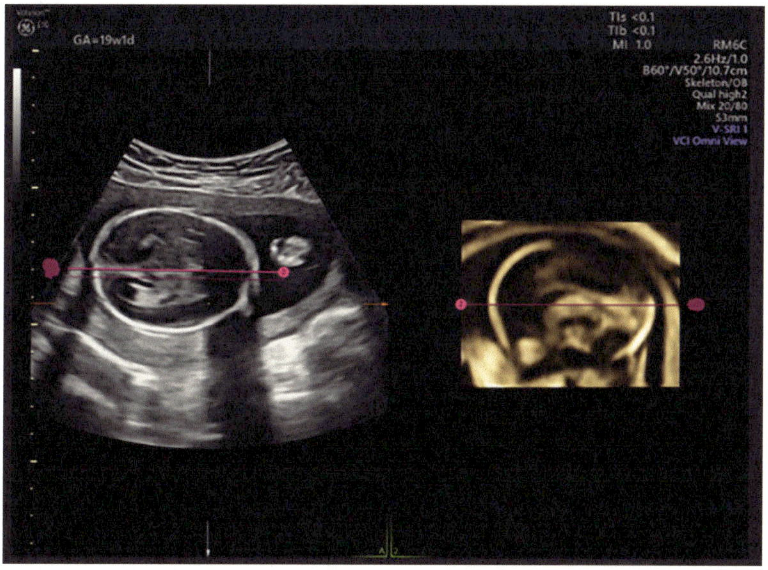

Figure 2.
VCI Omniview technique for the assessment of the corpus callosum at 19w1d based on initial axial transventricular plane (plane A) and a linear cut through the area of interest with corresponding virtual reconstruction of sagittal plane (plane B). Personal archive.

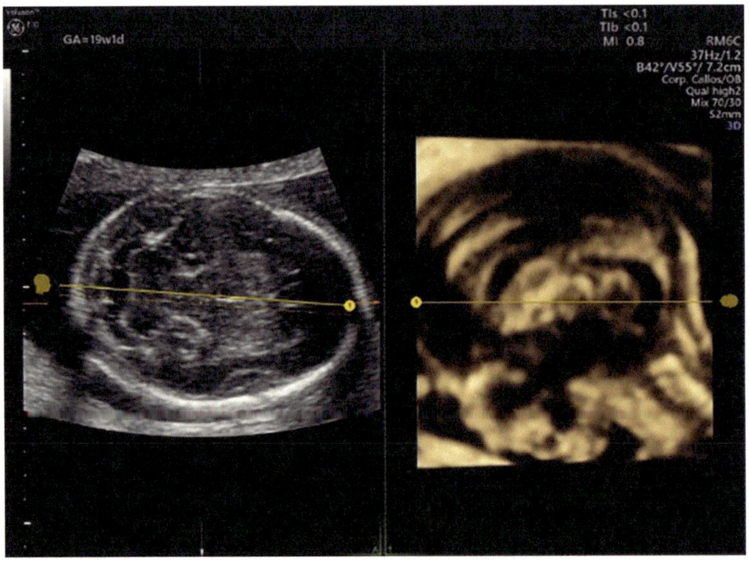

Figure 3.
VCI Omniview technique for the assessment of the corpus callosum at 19w1d based on initial axial transcerebellar plane (plane A) and a linear cut through the area of interest with corresponding virtual reconstruction of sagittal plane (plane B). Personal archive.

4. Other implications

The concept of "reorganization of the developing human brain" in the context of pathological conditions or lesions became of particular importance in the early 2000s when a study group reunited Nicolaides, Gratacos, Figueras and co. sought to evaluate the feasibility and reproducibility of volume segmentation of fetal intracranial structures using 3D ultrasound imaging [29]. Their results were in line with previous postnatal research, underlining the existence of selective growth restriction in certain brain regions which could disclose diminished cognitive function and delayed neurodevelopmental processes later in life [30]. The efficacy of a semiautomatic segmentation in 3D ultrasound volumes: Virtual Organ Computer-Aided Analysis (VOCAL) managed to show a reduction in the frontal and an increment in the thalamic volumes in fetuses with intrauterine growth restriction, compared with those appropriate for gestational age, matched by gestational age [29]. Later, the development of automatic segmentation of specific brain structures on 3D ultrasound volumes, addressed the need for manual delineation by an expert operator, centreing the cerebellum as a suitable anatomical landmark for intrauterine growth and health assessment [31, 32]. Calibration over movement, posture and balance is a hallmark of cerebellar function. There are some critical points to be addressed in the matter of cerebellar ultrasound volumetric study, which justify the peculiar interest of sonographers in this brain structure. First, the cerebellar volume is highly correlated with the gestational age and the transverse cerebellar diameter, and the specific organ segmentation provides the proper features for Dandy-Walker syndrome diagnosis; second, 2D ultrasound has several limitations regarding the measurements of lengths, contours or volumes of structures with an irregular shape as is the case of the cerebellum, and the manual segmentation is both time-consuming and inconsistent [33].

Benacerraf, a pioneer of ultrasound applications in prenatal diagnosis, presented an insightful use of volumetric ultrasound approaches in the detection and diagnosis of fetal brain anomalies. She emphasized the role of 3D scan used for the differential diagnosis of encephalocele, as well as for the reconstruction of the three orthogonal planes or for the tomographic cut involved in the diagnosis of septo-optic dysplasia, her work being in agreement with other ultrasound experts [19, 34].

Pooh et al. described the wide spectrum of volumetric ultrasound neuroimaging modes, highlighting the importance of unlimited offline analysis of the brain morphology, mentioning volume contrast imaging techniques (VCI) and HDlive silhouette imaging, at the same time questioning the role of fetal MRI in the diagnostic process [19, 20]. While at the beginning of 3D volumetric ultrasound use neurosonography was considered the centerpiece for fetal anomaly screening before 24 weeks of gestation and MRI after this gestational age, expert panels currently agree that these imagistic tools are complementary, MRI as a second-line investigation being relevant for diagnostic in only 7–15% of cases [3, 20].

Specifically for cases where CNS congenital defects are suspected, different ultrasound modes are more relevant than others, depending on the complexity of diagnostic criteria. For example, while ventriculomegaly can be easily depicted using axial views in 2D ultrasound which allows for accurate measurement of the enlarged atrial width in the lateral ventricles >10 mm, any structural impairment of corpus callosum, cerebellum or other posterior fossa structures still pose diagnostic challenges and require supplementary sagittal views, preferentially in multiplanar modes [20].

Corpus callosum and the cerebellum have been widely studied cerebral structures during intrauterine life, due to their relevance in normal development of motor, sensory and cognitive functions. These fundamental structures begin to develop early in the life of the embryo and their definitive functions are well established either at the end of the first year of postnatal life for the cerebellum or at the end of the second year of life for the corpus callosum [20, 35]. Although there have been almost 15 years since the fundamental principles of fetal neurosonography have been addressed by experts, there are still multiple limitations that encompass this practice: fetal brain development is a dynamic entity and can be susceptible to lesions later during pregnancy and in the postnatal life; parent counseling in cases of CNS anomalies involve diverse scenarios, from "nearly" normal neurological outcomes to severely impaired functions, depending on the complexity of the suspected condition [6, 20, 34]. The intricacy of prenatal CNS anomaly diagnosis goes even further, adding more knowledge to the core of the embryological development of all cerebral anatomical structures: ultrasound evaluation should be performed as a complete examination emerging from the latest international guidelines in the field and special consideration should be given to populational variability too. The most relevant example is that of corpus callosum evaluation, where its progressive morphological development – first of the anterior part and after of the posterior part, should be taken into account when suspecting potential hypoplasia after 20 weeks of gestation. Nevertheless, this adds to the fact that guidelines recommend rather a qualitative assessment than a quantitative one since a short, thin or thick corpus callosum is not necessarily synonymous with an abnormality of this cerebral structure [3, 19].

The rapid spread of fast volumetric ultrasound (4D) along with artificial intelligence technology in different medical fields can only represent the inception of a new era concerning innovations in imagistic diagnosis and therapy [12]. Precise motion tracking with 4D ultrasound is currently intensely studied and holds promising potential in prenatal screening and diagnosis. To fully understand the complexity of the brain, functional neuroimaging techniques could be of use in intrauterine life as well. Solutions could emerge from several investigations of functional ultrasound performed on rodents aiming to develop a method to image dynamic deep brain activation by directly measuring subtle cerebral blood volume changes [36]. Also, ongoing developments in the field of virtual reality enable experts to apply new research opportunities in the field of prenatal imaging as well: novel volumetric measurements based on segmentation of various parts of the fetal body at the end of the first trimester [37] possess the ability to add to an immersive body of knowledge with respect to adaptation mechanisms in early pregnancy which imply contextual adverse outcomes later in life.

To conclude, there is a remarkable multidirectional learning trajectory regarding ultrasound opportunities in prenatal diagnosis. The reliability of 2D ultrasound in obstetrics remains dependent on the skill and experience of the operator but there is evidence that both novice and expert interpretations of key biometric measurements of 3D volumetric datasets are highly reliable [38]. At the same time, the continuous search for domain shifting towards automatization in prenatal screening provides new evidence that with the use of system coordinates, it is now possible to automatically locate and segment the fetal brain and eye sockets in 2D and 3D images [39]. In contrast, based on economic and financial disparities resembling different healthcare systems, other researchers are focusing on reconstructing ultrasound volumes from 2D scans, without requiring extra equipment, since this method is widely used at the bedside; the results proved significant potential, at the same time promoting access for vulnerable populations of society to advanced monitoring in pregnancy [40, 41].

Acknowledgements

Acknowledgements to all pregnant patients admitted in the Obstetrics and Gynecology Department of "Sf. Pantelimon" Clinical Emergency Hospital for sharing their trust in their physicians.

No funding was received to assist with the preparation of this manuscript.

Conflict of interest

The author declares no conflict of interest.

Author details

Alexandra Matei
Department of Obstetrics and Gynecology, "Carol Davila" University of Medicine and Pharmacy, Bucharest, Romania

*Address all correspondence to: ale.matei@gmail.com

References

[1] Wang J, Nichols ES, Mueller ME, et al. Semi-automatic segmentation of the fetal brain from magnetic resonance imaging. Frontiers in Neuroscience. 2022;**16**:1027084. DOI: 10.3389/fnins.2022.1027084

[2] Malinger G, Paladini D, Haratz KK, et al. ISUOG practice guidelines (updated): Sonographic examination of the fetal central nervous system. Part 1: Performance of screening examination and indications for targeted neurosonography. Ultrasound in Obstetrics & Gynecology. 2020;**56**(3):476-484. DOI: 10.1002/uog.22145. Erratum in: Ultrasound Obstet Gynecol. 2022;60(4):591. doi: 10.1002/uog.26067

[3] Paladini D, Malinger G, Birnbaum R, et al. ISUOG practice guidelines (updated): Sonographic examination of the fetal central nervous system. Part 2: Performance of targeted neurosonography. Ultrasound in Obstetrics & Gynecology. 2021;**57**(4):661-671. DOI: 10.1002/uog.23616. Epub 2021 Mar 18. Erratum in: Ultrasound Obstet Gynecol. 2022;60(4):591. doi: 10.1002/uog.26067

[4] Salomon LJ, Alfirevic Z, Berghella V, et al. ISUOG practice guidelines (updated): Performance of the routine mid-trimester fetal ultrasound scan. Ultrasound in Obstetrics & Gynecology. 2022;**59**(6):840-856. DOI: 10.1002/uog.24888. Epub 2022 May 20. Erratum in: Ultrasound Obstet Gynecol. 2022;60(4):591. doi: 10.1002/uog.26067

[5] Ciceri T, Squarcina L, Giubergia A, et al. Review on deep learning fetal brain segmentation from magnetic resonance images. Artificial Intelligence in Medicine. 2023;**143**:102608. DOI: 10.1016/j.artmed.2023.102608

[6] Karl K, Kainer F, Heling KS, et al. Fetal neurosonography: Extended examination of the CNS in the fetus. Ultraschall in der Medizin. 2011;**32**(4):342-361. DOI: 10.1055/s-0031-1273463

[7] Herickhoff CD, Morgan MR, Broder JS, et al. Low-cost volumetric ultrasound by augmentation of 2D systems: Design and prototype. Ultrasonic Imaging. 2018;**40**(1):35-48. DOI: 10.1177/0161734617718528

[8] März K, Franz AM, Seitel A, et al. MITK-US: Real-time ultrasound support within MITK. International Journal of Computer Assisted Radiology and Surgery. 2014;**9**(3):411-420. DOI: 10.1007/s11548-013-0962-z

[9] Morgan MR, Broder JS, Dahl JJ, et al. Versatile low-cost volumetric 3-D ultrasound platform for existing clinical 2-D systems. IEEE Transactions on Medical Imaging. 2018;**37**(10):2248-2256. DOI: 10.1109/TMI.2018.2821901

[10] Park EY, Cai X, Foiret J, et al. Fast volumetric ultrasound facilitates high-resolution 3D mapping of tissue compartments. Science Advances. 2023;**9**(22):eadg8176. DOI: 10.1126/sciadv.adg8176

[11] Peng C, Cai Q, Chen M, et al. Recent advances in tracking devices for biomedical ultrasound imaging applications. Micromachines (Basel). 2022;**13**(11):1855. DOI: 10.3390/mi13111855

[12] Sprenger J, Bengs M, Gerlach S, et al. Systematic analysis of volumetric ultrasound parameters for markerless 4D motion tracking. International Journal of Computer Assisted Radiology

and Surgery. 2022;**17**(11):2131-2139. DOI: 10.1007/s11548-022-02665-5

[13] Yang X, Wang X, Wang Y, et al. Hybrid attention for automatic segmentation of whole fetal head in prenatal ultrasound volumes. Computer Methods and Programs in Biomedicine. 2020;**194**:105519. DOI: 10.1016/j.cmpb.2020.105519

[14] Yang X, Yu L, Li S, et al. Towards automated semantic segmentation in prenatal volumetric ultrasound. IEEE Transactions on Medical Imaging. 2019;**38**(1):180-193. DOI: 10.1109/TMI.2018.2858779

[15] Xie HN, Wang N, He M, et al. Using deep-learning algorithms to classify fetal brain ultrasound images as normal or abnormal. Ultrasound in Obstetrics & Gynecology. 2020;**56**(4):579-587. DOI: 10.1002/uog.21967

[16] Huang R, Namburete A, Noble A. Learning to segment key clinical anatomical structures in fetal neurosonography informed by a region-based descriptor. Journal of Medical Imaging (Bellingham). 2018;**5**(1):014007. DOI: 10.1117/1.JMI.5.1.014007

[17] Salomon LJ, Alfirevic Z, Bilardo CM, et al. ISUOG practice guidelines: Performance of first-trimester fetal ultrasound scan. Ultrasound in Obstetrics & Gynecology. 2013;**41**(1):102-113. DOI: 10.1002/uog.12342. Erratum in: Ultrasound Obstet Gynecol. 2013;41(2):240

[18] Chaoui R, Heling KS, Kainer F, et al. Fetale Neurosonografie mittels 3-dimensionaler multiplanarer Sonografie [Fetal neurosonography using 3-dimensional multiplanar sonography]. Zeitschrift für Geburtshilfe und Neonatologie. 2012;**216**(2):54-62. DOI: 10.1055/s-0032-1308960

[19] Paladini D, Volpe P. Ultrasound of Congenital Fetal Anomalies. Differential Diagnosis and Prognostic Indicators. 2nd ed. Boca Raton, FL: Taylor and Francis Group; 2014. pp. 1-95. Ebook ISBN: 9780429462450

[20] Lipa M, Pooh RK, Wielgoś M. Three-dimensional neurosonography - A novel field in fetal medicine. Ginekologia Polska. 2017;**88**(4):215-221. DOI: 10.5603/GP.a2017.0041

[21] The 11-13 weeks scan: Early diagnosis of fetal defects - acrania/anencephaly. Fetal Medicine Foundation Courses. Available from: https://courses.fetalmedicine.com/fmf/show/159?locale=en [Accessed: June 26, 2024]

[22] Ushakov F, Sacco A, Andreeva E, et al. Crash sign: New first-trimester sonographic marker of spina bifida. Ultrasound in Obstetrics & Gynecology. 2019;**54**(6):740-745. DOI: 10.1002/uog.20285

[23] Chang CH, Yu CH, Chang FM, et al. The assessment of normal fetal brain volume by 3-D ultrasound. Ultrasound in Medicine & Biology. 2003;**29**(9):1267-1272. DOI: 10.1016/s0301-5629(03)00989-x

[24] Chen HC, Tsai PY, Huang HH, et al. Registration-based segmentation of three-dimensional ultrasound images for quantitative measurement of fetal craniofacial structure. Ultrasound in Medicine & Biology. 2012;**38**(5):811-823. DOI: 10.1016/j.ultrasmedbio.2012.01.025

[25] Scott JA, Habas PA, Kim K, et al. Growth trajectories of the human fetal brain tissues estimated from 3D reconstructed in utero MRI. International Journal of Developmental Neuroscience. 2011;**29**(5):529-536. DOI: 10.1016/j.ijdevneu.2011.04.001

[26] Gholipour A, Estroff JA, Barnewolt CE, et al. Fetal brain volumetry through MRI volumetric reconstruction and segmentation. International Journal of Computer Assisted Radiology and Surgery. 2011;**6**(3):329-339. DOI: 10.1007/s11548-010-0512-x

[27] Yin H, Li Y. Diagnostic value of Omniview technique on the agenesis of corpus callosum. The Journal of Maternal-Fetal & Neonatal Medicine. 2019;**32**(22):3806-3811. DOI: 10.1080/14767058.2018.1472230

[28] Altmann R, Scharnreitner I, Scheier T, et al. Sonoembryology of the fetal posterior fossa at 11 + 3 to 13 + 6 gestational weeks on three-dimensional transvaginal ultrasound. Prenatal Diagnosis. 2016;**36**(8):731-737. DOI: 10.1002/pd.4852

[29] Benavides-Serralde A, Hernández-Andrade E, Fernández-Delgado J, et al. Three-dimensional sonographic calculation of the volume of intracranial structures in growth-restricted and appropriate-for-gestational age fetuses. Ultrasound in Obstetrics & Gynecology. 2009;**33**(5):530-537. DOI: 10.1002/uog.6343

[30] Tideman E, Marsál K, Ley D. Cognitive function in young adults following intrauterine growth restriction with abnormal fetal aortic blood flow. Ultrasound in Obstetrics & Gynecology. 2007;**29**(6):614-618. DOI: 10.1002/uog.4042

[31] Gutierrez, Becker B, Arambula Cosio F, Guzman Huerta ME, et al. Automatic segmentation of the cerebellum of fetuses on 3D ultrasound images, using a 3D point distribution model. In: Annu Int Conf IEEE (Institute of Electrical and Electronics Engineers) Eng Med Biol Soc. Buenos Aires, Argentina. 2010. pp. 4731-4734

[32] Gutiérrez-Becker B, Arámbula Cosío F, Guzmán Huerta ME, et al. Automatic segmentation of the fetal cerebellum on ultrasound volumes, using a 3D statistical shape model. Medical & Biological Engineering & Computing. 2013;**51**(9):1021-1030. DOI: 10.1007/s11517-013-1082-1

[33] Liu X, Yu J, Wang Y, et al. Automatic localization of the fetal cerebellum on 3D ultrasound volumes. Medical Physics. 2013;**40**(11):112902. DOI: 10.1118/1.4824058

[34] Doubilet PM, Benson CB, Benacerraf BR. Atlas of Ultrasound in Obstetrics and Gynecology: A Multimedia Reference, 3e. Philadelphia: Lippincott Williams & Wilkins, A Wolters Kluwer Business; 2019. pp. 3-109. ISBN: 9781496356055 [Accessed: September 24, 2024]

[35] Sadler TW. Langman's Medical Embryology. 12th ed. Baltimore: Lippincott Williams & Wilkins; 2012. pp. 285-317. ISBN: 9781451113426

[36] Rabut C, Correia M, Finel V, et al. 4D functional ultrasound imaging of whole-brain activity in rodents. Nature Methods. 2019;**16**(10):994-997. DOI: 10.1038/s41592-019-0572-y

[37] Wiertsema CJ, Erkamp JS, Mulders AGMGJ, et al. First trimester fetal proportion volumetric measurements using a virtual reality approach. Prenatal Diagnosis. 2021;**41**(7):868-876. DOI: 10.1002/pd.5947

[38] Salinaro JR, McNally PJ, Nickenig Vissoci JR, et al. A prospective blinded comparison of second trimester fetal measurements by expert and novice readers using low-cost novice-acquired 3D volumetric ultrasound. The Journal of Maternal-Fetal & Neonatal

Medicine. 2021;**34**(11):1805-1813. DOI: 10.1080/14767058.2019.1649390

[39] Namburete AIL, Xie W, Yaqub M, et al. Fully-automated alignment of 3D fetal brain ultrasound to a canonical reference space using multi-task learning. Medical Image Analysis. 2018;**46**:1-14. DOI: 10.1016/j.media.2018.02.006

[40] Yeung PH, Hesse LS, Aliasi M, et al. Sensorless volumetric reconstruction of fetal brain freehand ultrasound scans with deep implicit representation. Medical Image Analysis. 2024;**94**:103147. DOI: 10.1016/j.media.2024.103147

[41] Xie W, Namburete AIL. Sensorless volumetric reconstruction of fetal brain freehand ultrasound scans with deep implicit representation. Medical Image Analysis. 2024;**94**:103147. DOI: 10.1016/j.media.2024.103147

Chapter 3

Role of Ultrasound and Its Recent Applications in Diagnosing Fetal Malformations

Madhavi Latha Routhu

Abstract

Nowadays, ultrasound is widely used for diagnosing fetal abnormalities. For better outcomes, early diagnosis of fetal abnormalities are needed. It facilitates time for other investigations and counseling for management options. Some of the prenatally diagnosed significant structural abnormalities may result in termination of pregnancy. Most of the anomalies do not require any treatment. Some structural anomalies are associated with genetic conditions or may be due to infections. To know the rate of prenatal detection of the disorders by this modality is also essential. Recent ultrasound technical improvements like high-resolution linear transducers, radiant flow, 3D/4D technology, Spatiotemporal Image Correlation (STIC), Fetal HQ, and artificial intelligence enhance the evaluation of the fetal heart. This chapter will discuss the role of ultrasound and recent research for improving the detection rate of fetal abnormalities and the use of higher-end technical applications to improve diagnostic capability and functional analysis.

Keywords: ultrasound, genetic, syndrome, anomalies, fetal heart, fetal malformations

1. Introduction

Ultrasound is an essential tool for prenatal diagnosis because of its low cost, easy availability, non-invasive, no radiation, real-time display and excellent performance [1–3]. Prenatal ultrasound is a vital modality to evaluate fetal growth status and malformations. Recent research focuses on improving the first-trimester detection rate of fetal malformations. 64% of all significant cardiac anomalies in the low-risk population and around 80% in high-risk are diagnosed by performing a first-trimester fetal echo [4]. As per Syngelaki et al. [5], all cases of Acrania (**Figure 1**), alobar holoprosencephaly, large encephalocele, tricuspid or pulmonary atresia, pentology of cantrell, ectopia cardis, exomphalos, gastroschisis and body stalk anomaly are diagnosed on 11–13 weeks scan. The open spina bifida detection rate in the first trimester was improved from 15 to 59%, and significant cardiac defects from 5 to 35% [5]. This improvement is achieved by better quality ultrasound machines, standardized protocols, especially mid-sagittal sections of the brain for the posterior fossa, inclusion of color Doppler examination of four chamber views of the heart and outflow tracts and the transverse views of the face to demonstrate the upper lip and palate for diagnosing clefts [5].

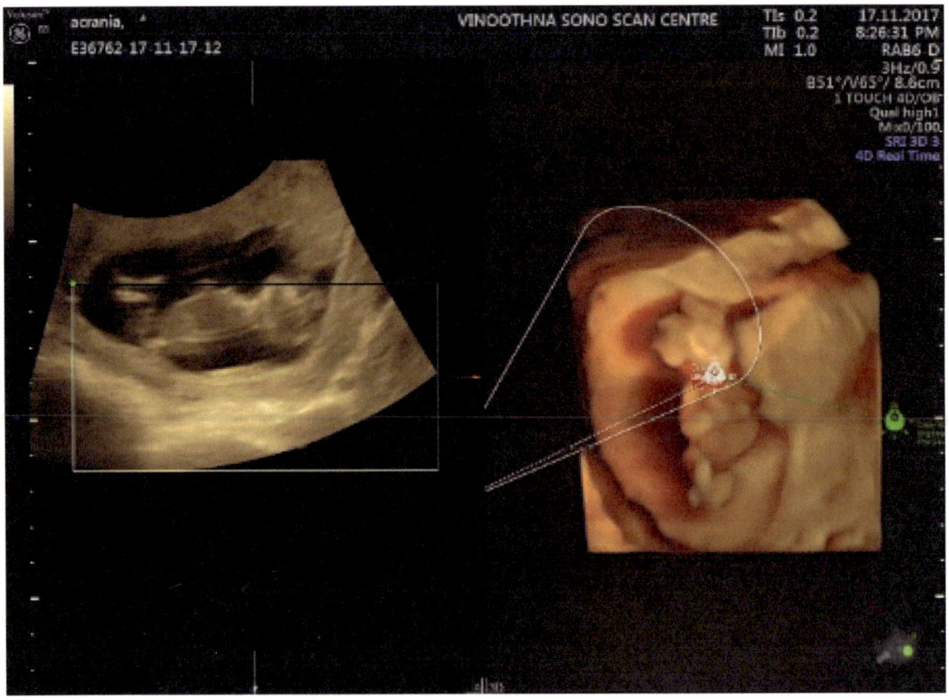

Figure 1.
Represents Acrania in HD live rendering.

The incidence of abnormalities first seen at 35–37 weeks was 0.5% [6]. At this examination, some of the cases of ovarian cysts, microcephaly, achondroplasia, dacrocystocele and hematocolpos were diagnosed first time with normal NT and second trimester ultrasound screening [6]. Detection of late third trimester other anomalies are cardiac lesions like 18% of VSDs, some of the Rhabdomyomas, mild pulmonary stenosis, mild aortic stenosis and aortic coarctation. Genitourinary anomalies are hydronephrosis and in GIT are Diaphragmatic hernias [6]. Detected only in advanced pregnancy are Cardiomyopathies, valvular stenosis, and tumors [7, 8].

2. Hints for detection of fetal anomalies and aneuploidy on ultrasonography

Not only ultrasound confirm intrauterine pregnancy, but it also detects the number of fetuses, where we can look for conjoined twins in monochorionic monoamniotic twins. The ultrasound signs for conjoined twins are the same relative positions in all views, direct opposition of the twins from each other, and inseparable skin contours that must be persistent and at the same anatomic level (**Figure 2**).

The first diagnostic ultrasound screening for aneuploidy is done at 11–13 + 6 weeks of pregnancy, where nuchal translucency is measured, and nasal bone ossification is confirmed.

The incidence of Downs syndrome (T21) is 1 in 750. The unossified nasal bone is detected in 60–70% of T21 fetuses and 55% in Edward syndrome (T18). According to

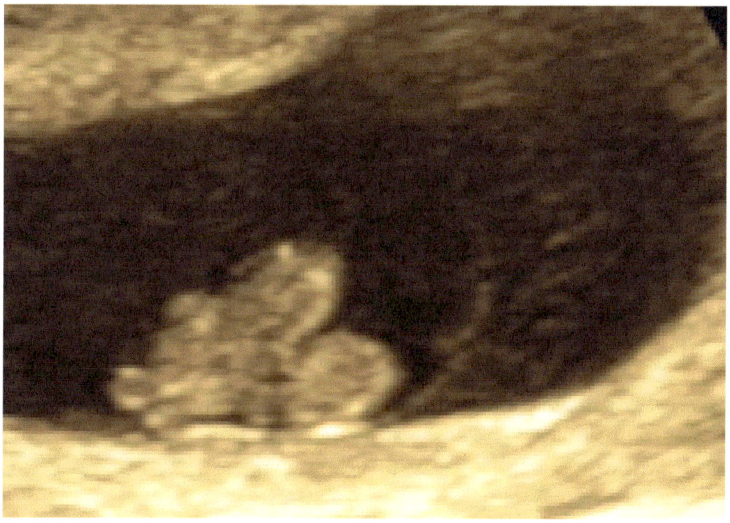

Figure 2.
Represents conjoined twins.

a meta-analysis, the unossified nasal bone is seen in 1.4% of normal fetuses. In Down syndrome, abnormal ductus venosus flow is noted in 80% of cases and short maxilla in 25% [9, 10]. In T18, early growth retardation and bradycardia were observed. Sometimes, it may be detected even at 11–13 + 6 weeks scan. 3% of healthy fetuses and 80% of T18 cases show a single umbilical artery [11]. Exomphalos 60% and 20% diaphragmatic hernia are associated with T18 in the first trimester. The other associated findings with T18 are strawberry-shaped head, choroid plexus cysts, absent corpus callosum, enlarged cisterna magna, fascial cleft, micrognathia, heart defects, oesophageal atresia, talipes, rocker bottom foot [12]. In Patau syndrome (trisomy 13), tachycardia is noted in 70% of cases [13]. Frequently associated common findings in T13 are holoprosencephaly, microcephaly, facial abnormalities, cardiac abnormalities, enlarged echogenic kidneys, megacystis, postaxial polydactyly and early growth retardation. Megacystis and holoprosencephaly are frequently detected [10]. Potentially identifiable significant fetal abnormalities in first trimester are early hydrops, anencephaly, alobar holoprosencephaly, Body stalk anomalies, ectopia cardis, large omphalocele, large gastroschisis, and megacystis.

The second level ultrasound screening is frequently performed at 18–20 weeks of gestation to look for congenital malformations, chromosomal anomalies and other syndromes, hence known as "genetic screening sonography.". The soft markers for aneuploidy include increased nuchal fold thickness, aberrant right subclavian artery (ARSA), echogenic bowel loops, echogenic intracardiac foci, mild lateral ventriculomegaly, mild hydronephrosis and short femur/Humerus. The other soft markers which are not included in risk calculation for aneuploidy are choroid plexus cysts, single umbilical artery, sandal gap toes, short ears, clinodactyly, increased iliac angle, duodenal atresia and small membranous VSD.

Structures to be examined in genetic sonography for screening are cranium, Face, spine, neck, heart, Lungs, diaphragm, stomach, abdominal wall, kidneys, bladder, and extremities.

3. Ultrasound findings in fetal anomalies

3.1 Central nervous system

Cranial anomalies are one of the most common congenital malformations. For routine screening of the fetal brain, there are three principal scan planes in axial view: 1. Trans thalamic view, 2. Trans ventricular view, 3. Trans cerebellar view. Any clues suggesting brain malformations need additional views (advanced neurography) in coronal (4 scan planes) and sagittal (3 scan planes) planes to improve the detection rate. The indication for detailed neuro sonography in the second trimester is the absence of cavum septum pallidum (CSP), ventriculomegaly, abnormal fourth ventricle, and cyst in the posterior fossa. Absent CSP may be seen as an isolated finding or in holoprosencephaly, corpus callosum agenesis, and septo optic dysplasia. If square-shaped, look for partial corpus callosal agenesis/callosal dysgenesis. CSP is wider in 22q11 deletion syndrome and in midline fascial clefts and is longer in the standard variant (dolichocephaly). Narrow CSP may be noted in the typical third trimester, hypoplastic corpus callosum and hydrocephalus [14, 15]. Ultrasound findings in alobar holoprosencephaly (**Figure 3**) are a cup-shaped mono ventricle with a dorsal cyst and snake under the skull sign. For alobar holoprosencephaly, the ultrasound detection rate is 100%, whereas for lobar and semi lobar holoprosencephaly, the detection rate is low; clues to detect these conditions are absent Corpus callosum, absent interhemispheric fissure anteriorly in lobar, presence of interhemispheric fissure (IHF) noted only between occipital lobes in semi lobar and absent IHF in the posterior frontal and parietal region in middle hemispheric variant. Ultrasound signs in complete corpus callosum agenesis showed that the direct sign on a midsagittal plane is absent corpus callosum (CC). The indirect signs are absent CSP, colpocephaly, steer horn or Viking helmet sign, three-line sign, indentation of lateral ventricle due to Probst bundles, cephalad extension of third ventricle, absent cingulate sulcus, sunburst sign, abnormal course of pericallosal artery. Partial agenesis of corpus callosum (**Figure 4**) the indirect signs are short and wide CSP and the CSP

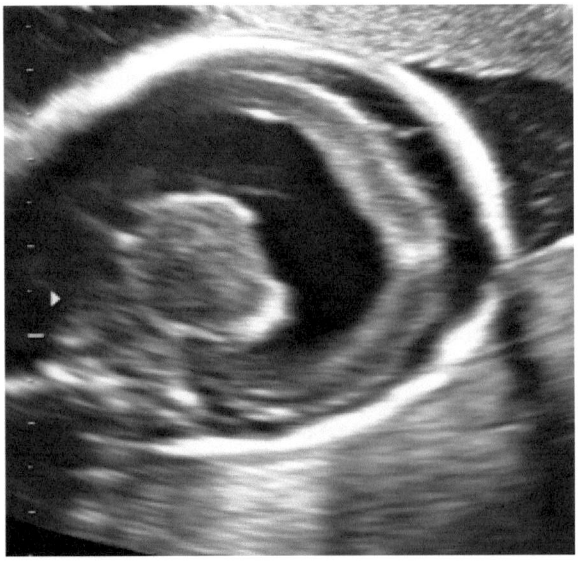

Figure 3.
Represents holoprocencephaly.

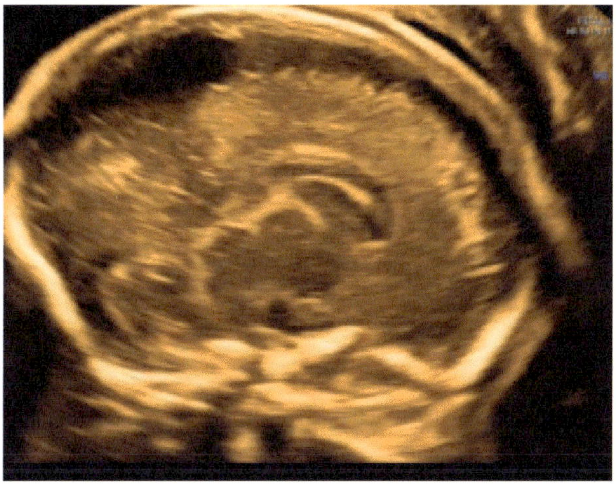

Figure 4.
Represents partial corpus callosal agenesis.

ratio is less than 1.5. Direct signs are absent splenium CC do not extend to overlie the tectal plate of the midbrain, absence of bulbosity of splenium, short cingulate sulcus and pericallosal artery is present only over the segment of the CC that is present. In the first trimester, Increased fluid in the posterior fossa – can be a transient finding, a subtle marker for aneuploidy, developing posterior fossa malformation, cerebellar hypoplasia and occipital encephalocele. Abnormal fourth ventricle index is the clue for Joubert syndrome, rhombencephalon synapsis, pontocerebellar hypoplasia and Walker-Warburg syndrome [16]. To differentiate posterior fossa malformation, look for length, AP diameter & area of vermis. Vermian diameter/BPD x 100 demonstrates the degree of rotation of vermis which is more in dandy walker malformation than dandy walker variant [17]. Clues for posterior fossa abnormalities are open fourth ventricle and cyst in the posterior fossa. Signs to detect Microcephaly are head circumference < -3SD, receding forehead, acoustic shadowing due to narrowed cranial sutures and foramen cranial distance < -2SD. In Lissencephaly shallow sylvian fissure forms figure of 8 and shallow or absent another sulcation are seen. In cobblestone complex (walker-Warburg syndrome) hyperechoic layer around the cerebral hemispheres, medial pseudo fusion, kinked (Z shaped) brainstem, nutcracker sign, delayed sulcation, hydrocephalus, ocular abnormality, low set ears are observed. In poly microgyria premature cerebral convexity sulcation appears as surface undulations. Schizencephaly the finding is trans mantle cleft lined by gray matter. Tuberous sclerosis-cardiac rhabdomyomas and cerebral tubers. Acrania anencephaly sequelae, Alobar holoprosencephaly, and large encephalocele are always detectable CNS abnormalities (**Table 1**).

3.2 Neural tube defects (NTD)

They are frequently reported anomaly. The incidence of NTD are 6.5–8.2/1000 live births. Anencephaly, encephalocele/meningocele and spina bifida are the most commonly detected NTDs [18–20]. Spina bifida are two types: 1. occulta: there is no protrusion and the affected area is covered with skin 2. cystica: presence of protrusion, and may be covered or not covered with skin. Meningocele contains meninges and cerebrospinal fluid whereas myelomeningocele contains meninges, cerebrospinal

Central Nervous System 11-14 Weeks 1% of all births	Always	Acrania
		Exencephaly
		Encephalocele
		Holoprosencephaly
	Sometimes	Spina bifida
		Hydrocephalus
		Blake's pouch cyst
		Dandy-Walker malformation
		Choroid plexus cysts
		Agenesis of the Corpus Callosum
		Cervical flexors
	Never	Infection microcephaly
		Lissencephaly
		Hemimegaloencephaly
		Scaphocephaly
		Schizencephaly
		Aneurysm of the vein of Galen
		Cerebellar hypoplasia
		Rhombencephalosynapsis
		Intracranial tumours/Lipomas
		Infection/ Haemorrhage/Dural Sinus Thrombosis

Table 1.
Represents detection of CNS anomalies in first trimester.

fluid and neural structures. Rachischisis/myeloschisis refers to a condition where the neural tube is completely exposed, without any covering of meninges or skin [21]. To improve the detection rate of NTD in first trimester, the indirect signs on sagittal view are non- visualization or obliteration of cisterna magna, non-visualization/ obliteration of intracranial translucency (**Figure 5**) and posterior shift of brain stem causing increased BS/BSOB ratio. On axial planes BPD <10%, expanded/dangling choroid plexus, posterior shift of aqueduct of Sylvius, crash sign, parallel cerebral peduncles are the potential early marker for NTD [22]. Lemon and Banana signs are the second trimester indirect signs for open NTD. Recent advances in technology, systemic protocol-based approach by using intracranial signs along with direct visualization of spine using higher frequency probe/trans vaginal approach can increase the detection rate of open neural tube defects by 50–90% [22]. Multiplanar or HD live rendering can improve the better crater visualization. Signs for closed spinal dysraphism are alteration in spinal curvature, missing vertebrae (atypical ossification of fetal spine), blunt ending spine with absence of sacral tapering and mass at the spine in sagittal plane [22]. On transverse plane are integrity of skin and soft tissue over the spine, defect over the spine and divergent pedicles, abnormal alignment of ribs and abnormal posturing of limbs and on coronal view. Inclusion of these signs increases the detection rate up to 60% [22]. The Sonographic features in diastematomyelia are

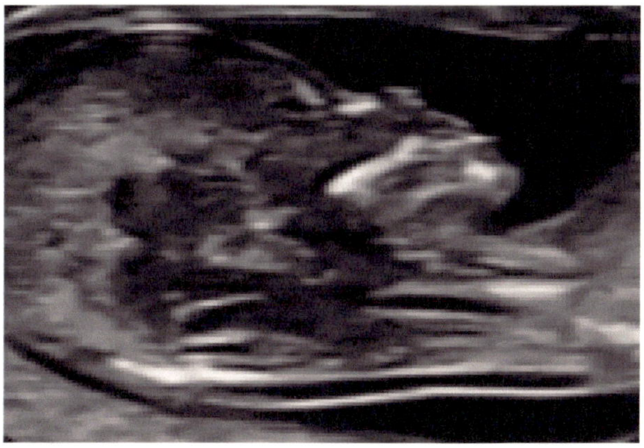

Figure 5.
Represents reduced intra craneal translucency in open NTD.

posterior ossification centres of vertebrae are widened, two hemicords with osseous/fibrous septum traversing the spinal canal and intact skin. In sacral dysgenesis the findings are abnormal sacral tapering (short spine with abrupt ending) and opposed iliac bones (shield sign) [22]. Wedge shaped vertebrae with subtle alignment alteration is seen in hemivertebrae.

3.3 Facial abnormalities

Due to the recent research by combining the mid-sagittal, axial and coronal views improves the detection rates of cleft lip and cleft palate from 5–35% [5]. The signs are (a) maxillary gap sign [23] (b) retronasal triangle view (**Figure 6**) [24] (c) Frontal space distance [25] increased in bilateral cleft lip with palate or micro/retrognathia (d) palatomaxillary diameter [26]. In retronasal triangle (RNT) plane complete absence of base indicates bilateral cleft palate, absent apex is unossified nasal bone. Complete absence of base of RNT with absent maxillary line suggests median cleft in holoprosencephaly. The absent superimposed line sign indicates cleft palate [27]. absent mandibular gap is micrognathia. In first trimester the palate is less curved and

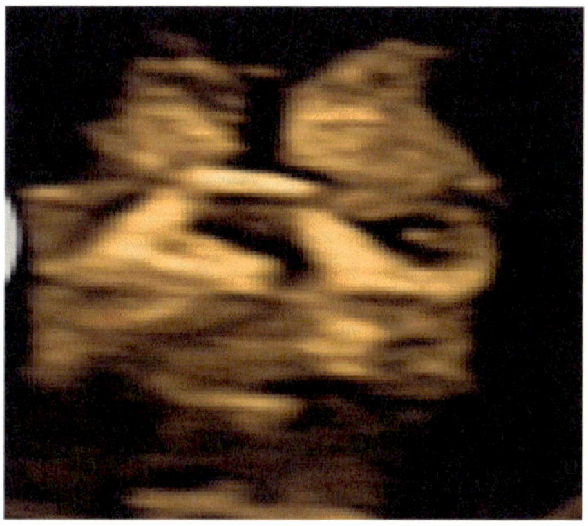

Figure 6.
Represents RNT in unilateral cleft lip and palate.

flat, so using 3D multiplanar imaging and tomographic ultrasound imaging (TUI) [27–29] improves the detection rate of cleft palate.

3.4 Congenital heart defects

Most common malformations are cardiac defects. The incidence rate is 1in 100 per live births [30]. The diagnostic planes to screen cardiac defects in first trimester are to look for situs, four chamber plane, four chamber color flow and 3VT view with color are needed. HD live depicting atrioventricular (AV) valve leaflets clearly [31]. The inclusion of four chamber and 3VT view in routine screening maximizes the detection of cardiac defects in all NT scans which aids in early detection of major cardiac anomalies [32]. The sensitivity for detection of major CHD of early cardiac screening in low-risk pregnancy is under 60% and majority of severe cardiac defects are detectable by use of simple scanning protocols [32].

Normal signs in fetal echo are x sign, tick sign, line and dot sign, anterior v sign, left v or posterior v sign. The clues for CHD in fetal echo are cardiac axis deviation and situs abnormalities [33]. Cardiac abnormalities with normal four chambers are transposition of great arteries, Tetralogy of fallot, pulmonary atresia with VSD, Double outlet right ventricle, Truncus arteriosus, mild ebsteins anomaly, small VSD/ASD, mild/moderate aortic/pulmonary stenosis, mild coarctation of aorta and partial anomalous pulmonary venous drainage hence inclusion of outflow tracts and 3VT views in screening procedure are needed. Hints for Total abnormal pulmonary venous return on 4chamber view are (**Figure** 7) smooth left atrium (LA), increased distance of left atrium to descending aorta, ventricular disproportion, dilated coronary sinus. On 3VT view presence of vertical vein noted. In atrio ventricular septal defect (AVSD) the ultrasound findings are four chamber shows absent Crux with color shows H sign (**Figure 8**) in five chamber view show elongated outflow tract (goose neck sign) [34]. Transposition of great artery (TGA) missed on prenatal diagnosis in more than 50% cases. In TGA the Left

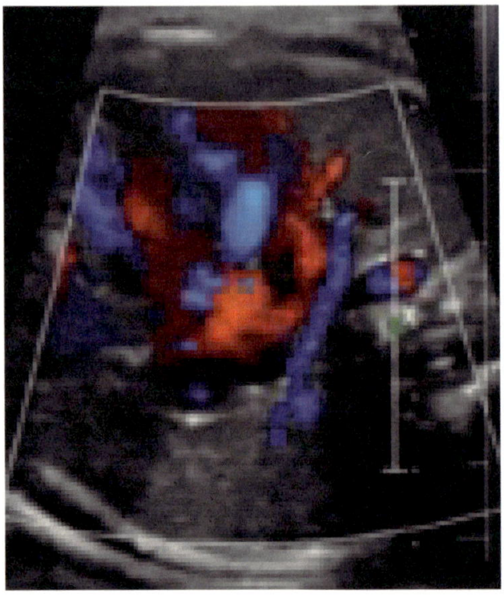

Figure 7.
Represents vertical vein in TAPVC.

ventricular out flow tract (LVOT) is always abnormal as it shows branching, two vessels on three Vessel view, Parallel great arteries (**Figure 9**) and most of the times 3VT views will be abnormal [34]. To rule out overriding in Conotruncal anomalies note the angle between the ventricular septum and ascending aorta, no blood from right ventricle to aorta and left ventricular outflow tract do not divide in transverse plane. The sign for overriding aorta is Y sign (**Figure 10**) [35] types of tetalogy of fallot (TOF) and associated malformations are depends on pulmonary artery (PA). PA forward flow in pink TOF, reverse flow in blue TOF, no flow in PA with presence of major aortopulmonary collateral arteries (MAPCA) confirms pulmonary atresia with ventricular septal defect (PAVSD), very large PA and its branches with regurgitation is absent pulmonary valve syndrome. TOF may be associated with right aortic arch, TOF associated with AVSD more commonly seen in heterotaxy, TOF with absent ductus arteriosus or it may also associate with abnormal origin of branch pulmonary artery [34].

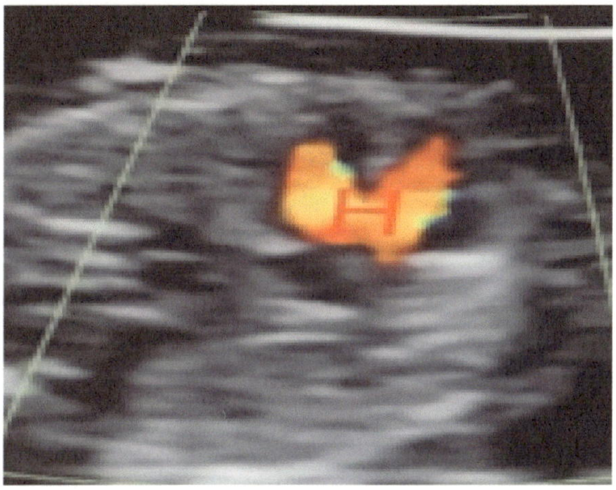

Figure 8.
Represents H sign in AVSD (atrioventricular septal defect).

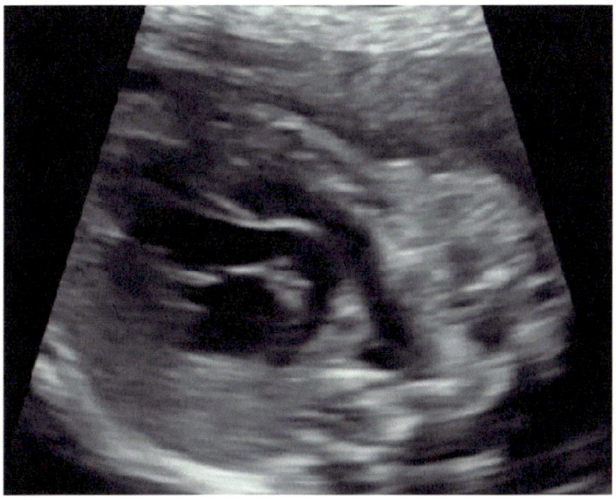

Figure 9.
Represents parallel great arteries in TGA.

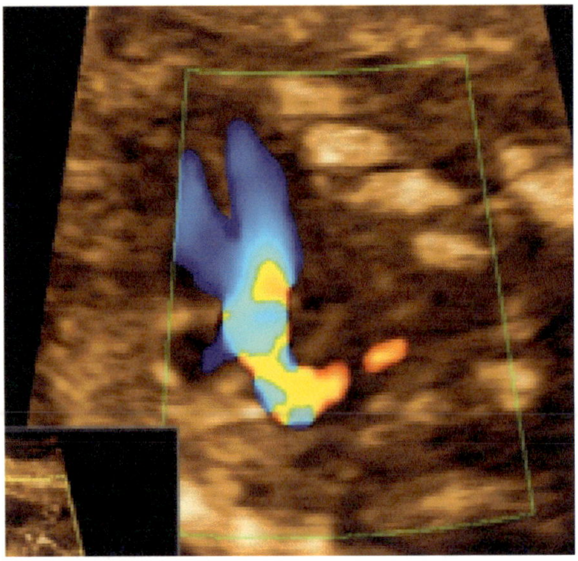

Figure 10.
Represents Y sign in overriding of Aorta.

3.5 Thoracic abnormalities

In left diaphragmatic hernia look for liver left up along with stomach in thorax. Bowel up in left diaphragmatic hernia the Superior Mesenteric Artery direction is toward thorax (**Figure 11**) [36]. High-frequency probe is useful in these cases to look for bowel peristalsis. LHR and quantitative lung index should be measured for the prognosis [36]. 3D used to calculate lung volume. Hyperechoic lung noted in congenital pulmonary airway malformations, bronchial atresia, congenital lobar emphysema, bronchopulmonary sequestration and neuroblastoma [37]. In bronchopulmonary sequestration-feeding artery from aorta and venous draining into azygos/hemiazygos vein.

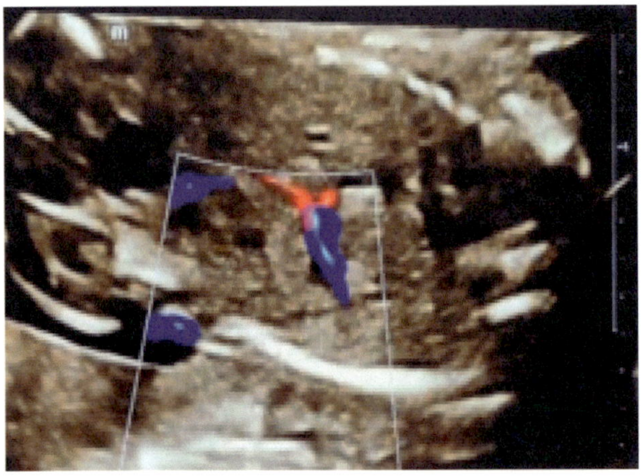

Figure 11.
Represents upward coursing of SMA in left diaphragmatic hernia.

3.6 Gastrointestinal anomalies

Sonographic findings of oesophageal atresia are polyhydramnios, persistently non visualized/small stomach, proximal esophageal pouch, dilated hypopharynx [38]. Persistently non visualized stomach is also seen in Arthrogryposis, cleft palate, micrognathia, Neckmass, CHAOS, epignathus, Anhydramnios and microgastria. Double bubble sign is seen in duodenal atresia. In jejunal atresia few dilated bowel loops, dilated stomach, polyhydramnios and there may be intrauterine growth retardation (IUGR) [39]. Ileal atresia – more dilated bowelloops, normal stomach and liquor. Perforation is more common finding. Ventral wall defects noted in Pentalogy of Cantrell, ectopia cardis, omphalocele, Gastroschisis, Bladder exstrophy, cloacal exstrophy, Limb body wall complex (**Figure 12**) and Amniotic band sequence (**Figure 13**) [40]. The differential diagnosis for ventral wall defect depends on (1) presence/absence of covering membrane, (2) cord insertion to defect, (3) depends on herniated organ, and (4) bowel appearance and associated anomalies [40].

3.7 Kidneys and bladder

Laid back adrenal sign is seen in renal agenesis. In Autosomal recessive polycystic kidney disease (ARPKD) – bilateral echogenic enlarged kidneys with loss of corticomedullary differentiation. Autosomal dominant polycystic kidneys – enlarged echogenic kidneys with exaggerated corticomedullary differentiation. Bladder exstrophy – persistent non filling of bladder, midline gut and lateral hemi bladder mucosal eversion appears as elephant trunk [41]. Causes of persistent non filled urinary bladder are bilateral renal agenesis, bilateral Multicystic dysplastic kidneys (MCDK), single kidney with MCDK, Unilateral MCDK with contralateral severe obstruction, ARPKD, cloacal exstrophy and rupture urinary bladder in lower urinary tract obstruction (LUTO). We can also predict renal function LUTO by doing visicocentesis for urine analysis depending on that fetal intervention may be offered [42].

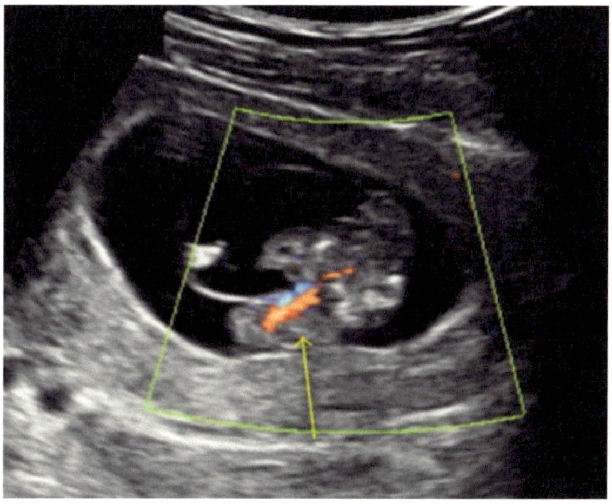

Figure 12.
Represents limb body wall complex.

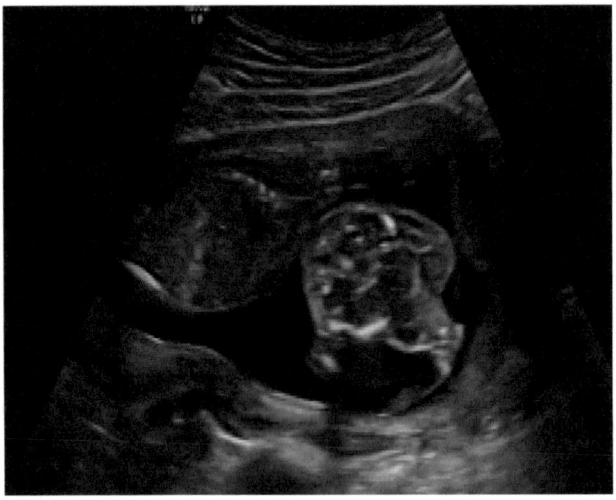

Figure 13.
Represents amniotic band syndrome.

3.8 Skeletal dysplasia (SD)

lethal skeletal dysplasia will have severe micromelia, narrow thorax, polyhydramnios and diagnosed early compare to non- lethal SD [43]. Ultrasound approaches for SD are length of long bones, mineralization, shape/form, fractures and femur foot length ratio. Lethal SD – Telephone receiver shape bones, platyspondyly, frontal bossing seen in thanatophoric dysplasia, fractures and unossified calvarium in osteogenesis imperfecta, Hypo mineralization of spine sparing the clavicle, hydrops and macrocrania is seen in Achondrogenesis. Narrow thorax with polydactyly in short rib polydactyly syndrome [43]. Bowed femur and tibia, hypoplastic scapula and ambiguous genitalia in campomelic dysplasia. Narrow thorax, echogenic kidneys and polydactyly in asphyxiating thoracic dystrophy. Non- lethal SD are Rhizomelia, macrocrania, frontal bossing trident hand are seen in achondroplasia. Mild narrow thorax, Acromesomelia, AVSD/ASD, polydactyly in Ellis van Creveld syndrome [43]. punctate epiphysis and binder facies in chondrodysplasia punctata, Acromesomelia and metaphyseal flaring in acromesomelic dysplasia. Hitch-hiker thumb and joint contractures in diastrophic dysplasia [43].

To optimize images, (i) select a high-frequency transducer wherever it is feasible. (ii) It is advisable to utilize linear and transvaginal high-resolution transducers. (iii) when doing transvaginal ultrasound utilize the other hand to manipulate the uterus. (iv) Combine harmonic imaging, compound imaging and speckle reduction. (v) Reduce the image sector. (vi) Image depth should be reduced. (vii) Zoom the region of interest to occupy around one-third to half of the ultrasound image. (vii) Utilize a single focal zone (ix) Adjust the dynamic range to achieve either a high or low contrast image. Adjust image resolution. (x) utilize cine loop to review the stored images [44].

4. Higher-end advanced applications in ultrasound machine

The International Society of Ultrasound in Obstetrics and Gynecology (ISUOG) released practice guidelines about the mid-trimester ultrasound scan [45]. For high-risk pregnancies the American Institute of Ultrasound in Medicine (AIUM) recently recommended detailed second and third trimester scans, as well as fetal echocardiography [46]. Guidelines for targeted neurosonography has been released by ISUOG recently [47, 48]. During the first-trimester ultrasonography, approximately half (50%) of significant structural abnormalities can be identified [49]. Conducting a routine scan at approximately 36 weeks of pregnancy can identify approximately 0.5% of fetal anomalies that were not previously recognized [6]. Utilizing a high-resolution ultrasound enables a detailed examination of first-trimester fetal anatomy, and enhances identification of even minor or subtle anomalies [50]. There have been numerous advancements in ultrasound technologies, such as high-resolution ultrasonography, linear transducer, radiant flow, three/four-dimensional (3D/4D) ultrasound, spatial and temporal image correlation (STIC), tomographic ultrasound imaging (TUI), omni view, speckle tracking of the fetal heart (HQ), and artificial intelligence for detecting small and subtle abnormalities.

4.1 High-resolution ultrasonography

Utilizing high-frequency transducer, harmonic imaging (HI), spatial compound imaging (SCI), and speckle reduction imaging (SRI) in high-resolution ultrasonography improves images and signal processing with minimal tissue penetration [50]. In HI by exploiting the non-linear propagation of ultrasound through the body tissues produces high-resolution images with minimal artifacts [50]. Tissue harmonic imaging (THI) enhances image quality by eliminating low-intensity echoes which clouds the image when the transducer's fundamental frequency is utilized. SCI, can effectively reduce angle-dependent artifacts by integrating several lines of sight into a single composite image. Utilizing SRI can diminish speckles for further enhancement of image resolution [50]. As per ISUOG guidelines it is helpful to utilize a high-frequency transducer for fetal echocardiogram to identify minor heart abnormalities. In high BMI women HI can enhance the imaging resolution during the third trimester. ISUOG suggests transvaginal approach in cephalic presentation for advanced neuro sonography [48]. In podalic and head in higher up position transabdominal high-frequency transducer (8–9 MHz) can be utilized for neuro sonography. High-frequency transducers can suitable for examining the spinal cord, conus medullaris (**Figure 14**) [48], and also to rule out Lens and laryngeal pathologies in suspected cases [50].

Advances in color flow mapping are high-definition radiant flow and slow flow (**Figure 15**) are employed to visualize vasculature with high and slow flow rates. The latest advancements in postprocessing techniques for gray scale and color Doppler greatly enhance the visualization of ultrasound images.

4.2 3D ultrasonography

On 2D imaging when mid-sagittal view of brain is not perfectly obtained a 3D neurosongram was recommended by ISUOG. 3D displays thicker 'slices' which increases the signal-to background noise ratio on all three planes thereby enhances image resolution. In addition, multiplanar imaging correlation allows the display of perfectly aligned views on all three orthogonal planes [48]. In some of the malformations like facial clefts, micrognathia, and club foot needs additional information which can be provided by 3D ultrasonography [51]. 3D Skeletal mode

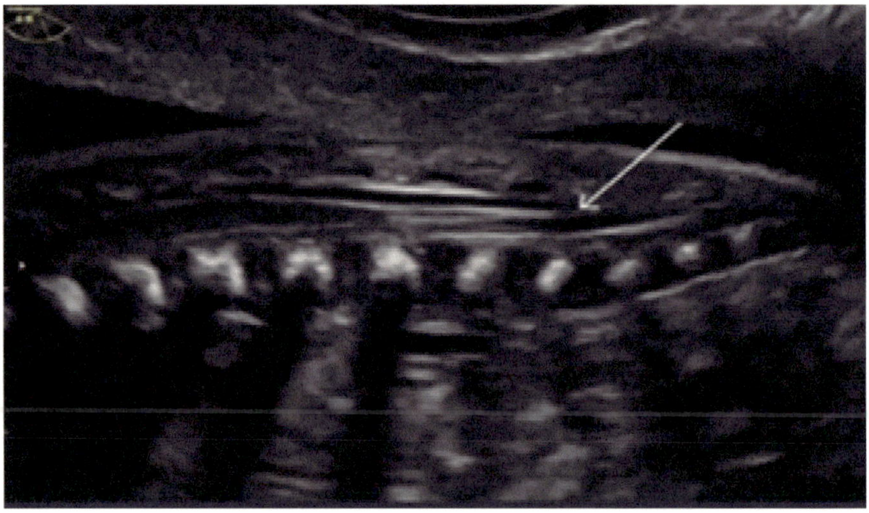

Figure 14.
Represents high resolution of sagittal plane of cauda equine.

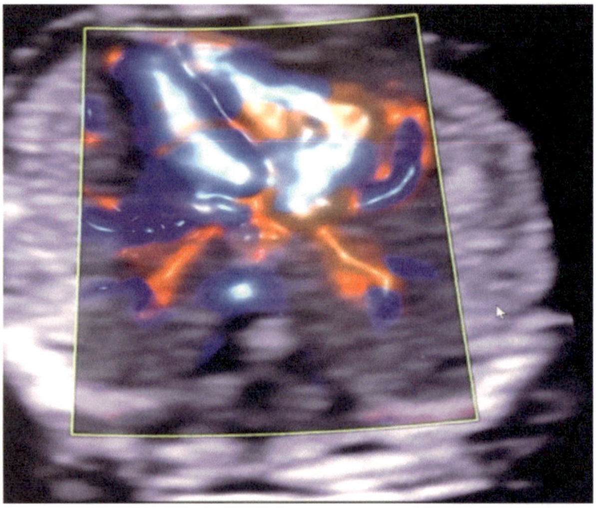

Figure 15.
Represents slow flow.

rendering can display skull, vertebrae, ribs, long bones and fingers (**Figure 16**) [52]. 3D ultrasound with multiplanar analysis and Crystal Vue rendering enable to visualize oesophagus which is challenging to see on routine 2D [53]. 3D ultrasound also aids in identifying ear and scapula abnormalities whenever needed. Most often dorsal spinal anomalies are very subtle and needs evaluation of ribs which is not accurately possible on 2D, hence 3D imaging is needed. Tomographic mode display of a 3D volume, which is able to show in one image several anatomic regions of the fetus. TUI enables the simultaneous display of both midsagittal and para sagittal sections in evaluation of palatine defects. Different types of clefts have a constant reproducible pattern in TUI [25].

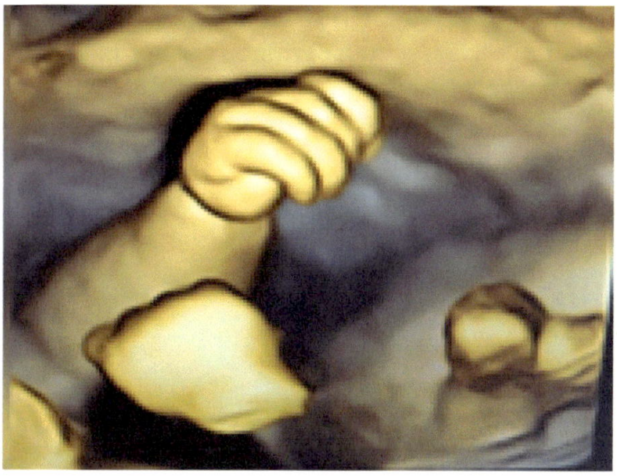

Figure 16.
Represents 3D rendering of fingers.

4.3 Spatiotemporal image correlation (STIC)

It acquires single 3D volume in a slow sweep with subsequent analysis of images in cine loop sequence in multiplanar/multi sliced format and rendered view which reduces the operation dependency of the ultrasound examination. STIC with color Doppler in glass-body mode (**Figure 17**) shows the anatomy of fetal heart and major vessels clearly [54]. With matrix probe we can rapidly acquire STIC volume, which reduces the motion artifact and facilitates live 4D display [54]. With matrix probe simultaneous examination in two orthogonal planes (biplane mode) can be done. Novel applications of STIC with electronic matrix transducer can acquire 3D volumes 4 times faster with enhanced resolution than conventional mechanical

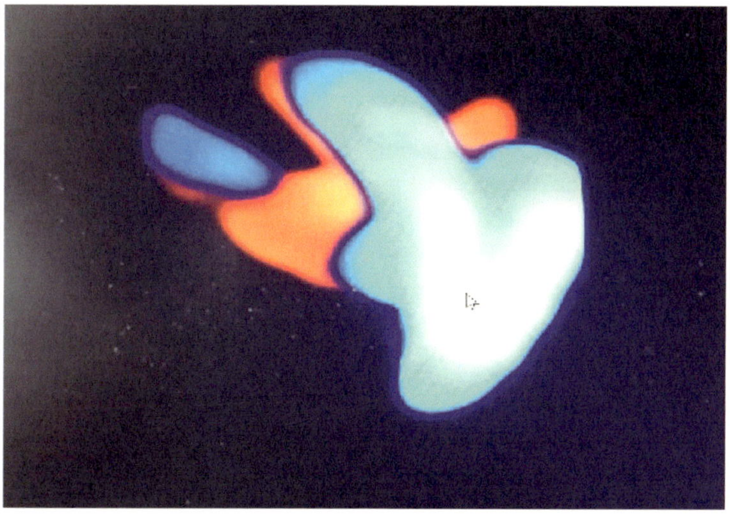

Figure 17.
Represents 4D STIC acquisition.

3D transducer. Electronic STIC (eSTIC) or rapid STIC can acquire a STIC volume within 2–3 s. 3D/4D allows to assess the cardiac volumes in systole and diastole [54]. Sono-VCAD for Volume Computer-Aided Diagnosis with a tomographic display of the retrieved planes [55] where the apical 4 chamber view has to be acquired. To confirm the volume orientation structures on the volume data sets are to be defined (septum, descending aorta, and others). The automation software then extracts the conventional diagnostic planes out of the volume and reduces the operator dependency [56].

4.4 3D printing

Recent researches in 3D technology allows the derived ultrasound data for 3D printing of whole fetuses [57] fetal face [58] or in cases of spina bifida where it can be beneficial for presurgical assessment [59]. With advances in STIC, a 3D printing of the fetal heart can be done [60] which can be easily downloaded from the machine as an STL (Standard Triangle Language) file, which can be seen on a personal computer using commonly available software and also used for 3D printing.

4.5 Fetal HQ

It is an innovative software which analyses cardiovascular system and allow the assessment of cardiac size, shape and contractility by utilizing speckle tracking at multiple points of the fetal heart [61]. The global sphericity index (SI) is a simple measurement of cardiac contractility, and it is equal to (end-diastolic mid-basal–apical length)/transverse length [62]. The sphericity index is calculated for each of the 24 end-diastolic transverse segments, which are located from the base to the apex of each ventricle as well as the end-diastolic mid-basal–apical length [61]. The SI for each segment was independent of gestational age and fetal biometry [62]. This index value is abnormal with cardiac chamber asymmetry like coarctation of aorta and pulmonary stenosis [61]. High risk of perinatal complications and childhood cardiovascular diseases are associated with abnormal SI values [63].

4.6 Artificial intelligence (AI)

AI has been increasingly utilized in prenatal ultrasonography in recent years, mostly for the purpose of recognizing standard planes, taking biometric measurements, and assisting in the detection of anomalies. AI models regularly used in medical imaging are: Convolutional neural network, U-Net and recurrent neural network. Machine learning is a subfield of AI that involves using data to learn and generate predictions or draw conclusions about new data, with the help of guidance [64]. Despite the standard application of United States, it might be difficult to obtain accurate readings in certain situations, like maternal obesity, motion blurring, missing borders, acoustic shadow, speckle noise, and a low signal-to-noise ratio [65]. AI applied on 2D images enables automatic computation of fetal biometry.

Deep learning is a sophisticated form of machine learning, uses artificial neural networks which connect through multiple synapses to exchange data with each other resembling the arrangement of neurons in the brain for analysing medical images closest to clinical application [66]. This complex algorithmic AI software is now being utilized in medicine to evaluate massive volumes of data, which can help prevent, diagnose and monitor patients' diseases. AI reduces the scanning time and

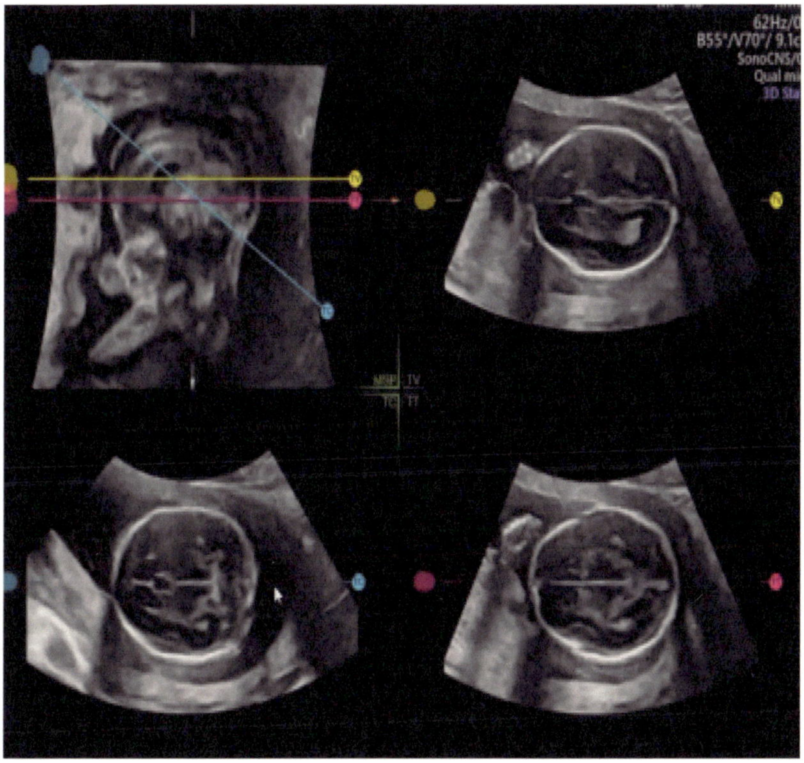

Figure 18.
Represents Sono CNS.

work-related musculoskeletal fatigue [67]. Sono NT automatically identifies and measures NT in mid-sagittal section [68]. In Sono CNS by applying AI on 3D volume of fetal head can auto calculate the CNS biometry (**Figure 18**) [69]. Sono-VCAD applied on STIC volume can navigate cardiac planes [70].

5. Discussion

Fetal malformation diagnosis depends on many factors like expertise &experience, machine and man, fetal age &maternal weight, interest & intellect And system involved and systemic approach. The overall prenatal detection rate of ultrasound screening with and without chromosomal anomalies was 57% [71], whereas only associated with chromosomal anomalies the detection rate was high approximately 88–93%. Without chromosomal anomalies ranged from 48 to 53% [71]. As per J M Carrera et al. between 1970 and 1991 fetal anomalies were diagnosed antenatally in 78.33% in routine ultrasound screening (**Table 2**) [72]. High-resolution ultrasonography can aid in the precise diagnosis of fetal echocardiography and targeted neurosonography in high-risk pregnancies [50]. Utilizing radiant flow can enhance the visualization of complex cardiac and vascular malformations. The use of 3D/4D ultrasound assist in prenatal diagnosis and counseling. High frequency transducer improves the diagnostic accuracy of some anomalies. Speckle tracking of the fetal heart enables evaluation of fetal heart morphology, dimensions, and contractility [50]. AI aids in recognizing accurate sectional planes and auto calculate the biometry, thereby decreasing the operator dependency and scan time [50].

Ultra sound fetal malformation		
Detection rate	**Frequency of anomaly**	**Earliest diagnosed malformations**
1970–74:19.75%	Urinary Tract: 22.86%	Thoracoabdominal wall:81.08%
1990–91:96.33%	Head and neck: 18.68%	Urinary Tract (70.83%)
	Musculoskeletal: 8.64%	Diaphragm 70.83%
	Heart anomalies: 7.35%	
	Gastrointestinal 7.35%	

Table 2.
Represents Journey of detection of malformation on routine prenatal ultra sound screening.

Although biochemical markers are sensitive to diagnose aneuploidy especially Downs syndrome, gestational age is an important parameter as the levels of markers depends on gestational age. For risk stratification nuchal translucency measurement is needed along with double marker. For estimation of accurate gestational age and measurement of nuchal translucency ultrasound is needed. By diagnosing structural defects on prenatal ultrasound condition can be better explained and easily convincible to the parents by direct demonstration of fetal images for further management options. Biochemical markers and ultrasound complement each other in aneuploidy screening [73].

6. Conclusion

Utilizing standard anatomical protocol improves the sensitivity of screening for all anomalies. International protocols with traditional anatomical views should be developed and introduced to optimize fetal anomaly detection. If you detect one anomaly, search for any additional related anomalies. Applying above mentioned recent technical applications and ultrasound signs will vastly improve the sensitivity of ultrasound in detecting anomalies in future.

Acknowledgements

The author wishes to express gratitude to Dr. B.S. Ramamurthy, Dr. Lakshmy Selvaraj for the source of information. Author also wants to wish thanks to Dr. Srujana, Dr. Hafeezuddin Dr. Sridevi and other colleagues of Radiology Department MGM hospital and also to Dr. G. Krishna, VRDL, Kakatiya Medical College, Warangal.

Author details

Madhavi Latha Routhu
Department of Radiology, MGM Hospital, Warangal, Telangana, India

*Address all correspondence to: madhaviradiologist@gmail.com

References

[1] Yang X, Wang X, Wang Y, Dou H, Li S, Wen H, et al. Hybrid attention for automatic segmentation of whole fetal head in prenatal ultrasound volumes. Computer Methods and Programs in Biomedicine. 2020;**194**:105519

[2] Oghli MG, Shabanzadeh A, Moradi S, Sirjani N, Gerami R, Ghaderi P, et al. Automatic fetal biometry prediction using a novel deep convolutional network architecture. Physica Medica. 2021;**88**:127-137

[3] Akkus Z, Cai J, Boonrod A, Zeinoddini A, Weston AD, Philbrick KA, et al. A survey of deep-learning applications in ultrasound: Artificial intelligence–powered ultrasound for improving clinical workflow. Journal of the American College of Radiology. 2019;**16**(9):1318-1328

[4] Karim JN, Bradburn E, Roberts N, Papageorghiou AT, ACCEPTS Study, Papageorghiou AT, et al. First-trimester ultrasound detection of fetal heart anomalies: Systematic review and meta-analysis. Ultrasound in Obstetrics & Gynecology. 2022;**59**(1):11-25

[5] Syngelaki A, Hammami A, Bower S, Zidere V, Akolekar R, Nicolaides KH. Diagnosis of fetal non-chromosomal abnormalities on routine ultrasound examination at 11-13 weeks' gestation. Ultrasound in Obstetrics & Gynecology. 2019;**54**(4):468-476

[6] Ficara A, Syngelaki A, Hammami A, Akolekar R, Nicolaides KH. Value of routine ultrasound examination at 35-37 weeks' gestation in diagnosis of fetal abnormalities. Ultrasound in Obstetrics & Gynecology. 2020;**55**(1):75-80

[7] Martinez D. Prenatal ultrasound diagnosis of congenital lung lesions. Pediatric Pulmonology. 2001;**32** (Suppl. 23):120-121

[8] Cunningham FG, Leveno KJ, Bloom SL, Hauth JC, Rouse DJ, Spong CY. Fetal imaging. In: Williams Obstetrics. New York: The McGraw-Hill Companies Inc; 2010. pp. 349-371

[9] Nicolaides KH. Screening for fetal aneuploidies at 11 to 13 weeks. Prenatal Diagnosis. 2011;**31**:7-15

[10] Nicolaides KH. The 11-13+6 Weeks Scan. London: Fetal Medicine Foundation; 2004

[11] Rembouskos G, Cicero S, Longo D, Sacchini C, Nicolaides KH. Single umbilical artery at 11-14 weeks: Relation to chromosomal defects. Ultrasound in Obstetrics & Gynecology. 2003;**22**:567-570

[12] Pilu G, Nicolaides KH, Meizner I, Romero R. Waldo Sepulveda prenatal diagnosis of fetal anomalies ultrasound in obstetrics and gynaecology. European Practice in Gynaecology and Obstetrics. 2009:157-208. DOI: 10.1016/B978-0-444-51829-3.00010-6

[13] Liao AW, Snijders R, Geerts L, Spencer K, Nicolaides KH. Fetal heart rate in chromosomally abnormal fetuses. Ultrasound in Obstetrics and Gynecology: The Official Journal of the International Society of Ultrasound in Obstetrics and Gynecology. 2000;**16**(7):610-613

[14] Chaoui R, Heling KS, Zhao Y, Sinkovskaya E, Abuhamad A, Karl K. Dilated cavum septi pellucidi in fetuses with microdeletion 22q11. Prenatal Diagnosis. 2016;**36**(10):911-915

[15] Karl K, Esser T, Heling KS, Chaoui R. CSP ratio: A marker for partial agenesis of the fetal corpus callosum. Ultrasound in Obstetrics & Gynecology. 2017;**50**:336-341

[16] Haratz KK, Shulevitz SL, Leibovitz Z, Lev D, Shalev J, Tomarkin M, et al. Fourth ventricle index: Sonographic marker for severe fetal vermian dysgenesis/agenesis. Ultrasound in Obstetrics & Gynecology. 2019;**53**:390-395

[17] Paladini D, Volpe P. Posterior fossa and vermian morphometry in the characterization of fetal cerebellar abnormalities: A prospective three-dimensional ultrasound study. Ultrasound in Obstetrics and Gynecology: The Official Journal of the International Society of Ultrasound in Obstetrics and Gynecology. 2006;**27**(5):482-489

[18] Levi S, Hyjazi Y, Schaapst JP, Defoort P, Coulon R, Buekens P. Sensitivity and specificity of routine antenatal screening for congenital anomalies by ultrasound: The Belgian multicentric study. Ultrasound in Obstetrics and Gynecology: The Official Journal of the International Society of Ultrasound in Obstetrics and Gynecology. 1991;**1**(2):102-110

[19] Tóth Z, Papp Z. Szülészet-nőgyógyászati Ultrahang-diagnosztika. Budapest, Hungary: White Golden; 2001. 508 p

[20] Papp Z, Borsos A, Kápolnai I, Kovács L, Mayer Á, Paulin F, et al. A szülészet-nőgyógyászat tankönyve. Budapest: Semmelweis Kiadó; 2007

[21] Buschbacher RM. Rehabilitation medicine quick reference. Spine. 2010:66-67

[22] Paoletti D, Robertson M, Sia SB. A sonographic approach to prenatal classification of congenital spine anomalies. Australasian Journal of Ultrasound in Medicine. 2014;**17**(1):20-37

[23] Chaoui R, Orosz G, Heling KS, Sarut-Lopez A, Nicolaides KH. Maxillary gap at 11-13 weeks' gestation: Marker of cleft lip and palate. Ultrasound in Obstetrics & Gynecology. 2015;**46**(6):665-669

[24] Sepulveda W, Wong AE, Martinez-Ten P, Perez-Pedregosa J. Retronasal triangle: A sonographic landmark for the screening of cleft palate in the first trimester. Ultrasound in Obstetrics and Gynecology: The Official Journal of the International Society of Ultrasound in Obstetrics and Gynecology. 2010;**35**(1):7-13

[25] Hoopmann M, Sonek J, Esser T, Bilardo CM, Wagner P, Abele H, et al. Frontal space distance in facial clefts and retrognathia at 11-13 weeks' gestation. Ultrasound in Obstetrics & Gynecology. 2016;**48**(2):171-176

[26] Lachmann R, Schilling U, Bru¨ckmann D, Weichert A, Bru¨ckmann A. Isolated cleft lip and palate: Maxillary gap sign and palatino-maxillary diameter at 11-13 weeks. Fetal Diagnosis and Therapy. 2018;**44**(4):241-246

[27] Lakshmy SR, Rose N, Masilamani P, Umapathy S, Ziyaulla T. Absent 'superimposed-line'sign: Novel marker in early diagnosis of cleft of fetal secondary palate. Ultrasound in Obstetrics & Gynecology. 2020;**56**(6):906-915

[28] Lakshmy SR, Deepa S, Rose N, Mookan S, Agnees J. First-trimester sonographic evaluation of palatine clefts: A novel diagnostic approach. Journal of Ultrasound in Medicine. 2017;**36**(7):1397-1414

[29] Lakshmy SR, Rose N, Masilamani P, Umapathy S, Ziyaulla T. Role of TUI in first trimester evaluation of palate. Journal of Fetal Medicine. 2019;**6**(3):113-121

[30] Hoffman JI, Kaplan S. The incidence of congenital heart disease. Journal of the American college of cardiology. 2002;**39**(12):1890-1900

[31] Lakshmy SR, Jain B, Rose N. Role of HD live in imaging the fetal heart. Journal of Ultrasound in Medicine. 2017;**36**(6):1267-1278

[32] Bottelli L, Franzè V, Tuo G, Buffelli F, Paladini D. Prenatal detection of congenital heart disease at 12-13 gestational weeks: Detailed analysis of false-negative cases. Ultrasound in Obstetrics & Gynecology. 2023;**61**(5):577-586

[33] Sinkovskaya ES, Chaoui R, Karl K, Andreeva E, Zhuchenko L, Abuhamad AZ. Fetal cardiac axis and congenital heart defects in early gestation. Obstetrics & Gynecology. 2015;**125**(2):453-460

[34] Bravo-Valenzuela NJ, Peixoto AB, Júnior EA. Prenatal diagnosis of congenital heart disease: A review of current knowledge. Indian Heart Journal. 2018;**70**(1):150-164

[35] Chaoui R, McEwing R. Three cross-sectional planes for fetal color Doppler echocardiography. Ultrasound in Obstetrics and Gynecology: The Official Journal of the International Society of Ultrasound in Obstetrics and Gynecology. 2003;**21**(1):81-93

[36] Lakshmy RS, Agnees J, Rose N. The upturned superior mesenteric artery sign for first-trimester detection of congenital diaphragmatic hernia and Omphalocele. Journal of Ultrasound in Medicine. 2017;**36**(3):583-592

[37] King SJ, Pilling DW, Walkinshaw S. Fetal echogenic lung lesions: Prenatal ultrasound diagnosis and outcome. Pediatric Radiology. 1995;**25**:208-210

[38] Pardy C, D'Antonio F, Khalil A, Giuliani S. Prenatal detection of esophageal atresia: A systematic review and meta-analysis. Acta obstetricia et gynecologica Scandinavica. 2019;**98**(6):689-699

[39] Apostolia G, Athanasios Z, Lampros P, Eirini M, Konstantinos Z, George M. Prenatal diagnosis of fetal jejunal atresia: A case report. Cureus. 2021;**13**(10):18947

[40] Atasever S, Azginoglu N, Terzi DS, Terzi R. A comprehensive survey of deep learning research on medical image analysis with focus on transfer learning. Clinical Imaging. 2023;**94**:18-41

[41] Gearhart JP, Ben-Chaim J, Jeffs RD, Sanders RC. Criteria for the prenatal diagnosis of classic bladder exstrophy. Obstetrics & Gynecology. 1995;**85**(6):961-964

[42] Haeri S. Fetal lower urinary tract obstruction (LUTO): A practical review for providers. Maternal Health, Neonatology and Perinatology. 2015;**1**:1-6

[43] Schramm T, Gloning KP, Minderer S, Daumer-Haas C, Hörtnagel K, Nerlich A, et al. Prenatal sonographic diagnosis of skeletal dysplasias. Ultrasound in Obstetrics and Gynecology: The Official Journal of the International Society of Ultrasound in Obstetrics and Gynecology. 2009;**34**(2):160-170

[44] Zander D, Hüske S, Hoffmann B, Cui XW, Dong Y, Lim A, et al. Ultrasound image optimization ("knobology"): B-mode. Ultrasound International Open. 2020;**6**(01):E14-E24

[45] Salomon LJ, Alfirevic Z, Berghella V, Bilardo C, Hernandez-Andrade E, Johnsen SL, et al. Practice guidelines for performance of the routine mid-trimester fetal ultrasound scan. Ultrasound in Obstetrics & Gynecology. 2011;**37**(1):116-126

[46] Carvalho JS, Axt-Fliedner R, Chaoui R, Copel JA, Cuneo BF, Goff D, et al. ISUOG practice guidelines (updated): Fetal cardiac screening.

Ultrasound in Obstetrics & Gynecology. 2023;**61**(6):788-803

[47] Malinger G, Paladini D, Haratz KK, Monteagudo A, Pilu GL, Timor-Tritsch IE. ISUOG practice guidelines (updated): Sonographic examination of the fetal central nervous system. Part 1: Performance of screening examination and indications for targeted neurosonography. Ultrasound in Obstetrics & Gynecology. 2020;**56**:476-484

[48] Paladini D, Malinger G, Birnbaum R, Monteagudo A, Pilu G, Salomon LJ, et al. ISUOG practice guidelines (updated): Sonographic examination of the fetal central nervous system. Part 2: Performance of targeted neurosonography. Ultrasound in Obstetrics & Gynecology. 2021;**57**:661-671

[49] Kenkhuis MJ, Bakker M, Bardi F, Fontanella F, Bakker MK, Fleurke-Rozema JH, et al. Effectiveness of 12-13-week scan for early diagnosis of fetal congenital anomalies in the cell-free DNA era. Ultrasound in Obstetrics & Gynecology. 2018;**51**(4):463-469

[50] Leung KY. Applications of advanced ultrasound technology in obstetrics. Diagnostics. 2021;**11**(7):1217

[51] Edwards L, Hui L. First and second trimester screening for fetal structural anomalies. Seminars in Fetal and Neonatal Medicine. 2018;**23**(2):102-111

[52] Tutschek B, Blaas HK, Abramowicz J, Baba K, Deng J, Lee W, et al. Three-dimensional ultrasound imaging of the fetal skull and face. Ultrasound in obstetrics & gynecology: The Official Journal of the International Society of Ultrasound in Obstetrics and Gynecology. 2017;**50**(1):7-16

[53] Dall'Asta A, Grisolia G, Nanni M, Volpe N, Schera GB, Frusca T, et al. Sonographic demonstration of fetal esophagus using three-dimensional ultrasound imaging. Ultrasound in Obstetrics & Gynecology. 2019;**54**(6):746-751

[54] Chaoui R, Abuhamad A, Martins J, Heling KS. Recent development in three and four dimension fetal echocardiography. Fetal Diagnosis and Therapy. 2020;**47**(5):345-353

[55] Abuhamad A, Falkensammer P, Reichartseder F, Zhao Y. Automated retrieval of standard diagnostic fetal cardiac ultrasound planes in the second trimester of pregnancy: A prospective evaluation of software. Ultrasound in Obstetrics and Gynecology: The Official Journal of the International Society of Ultrasound in Obstetrics and Gynecology. 2008;**31**(1):30-36

[56] Yeo R. Intelligent navigation to improve obstetrical sonography ultrasound. Obstetrics and Gynecology. 2016;**47**(4):403-409

[57] Tutschek B, Blaas HG. A human embryo in the palm of your hand. Ultrasound in Obstetrics & Gynecology. 2017;**50**(4):539-540

[58] Coté JJ, Badura-Brack AS, Walters RW, Dubay NG, Bredehoeft MR. Randomized controlled trial of the effects of 3D-printed models and 3D ultrasonography on maternal–fetal attachment. Journal of Obstetric, Gynecologic & Neonatal Nursing. 2020;**49**(2):190-199

[59] Miller JL, Ahn ES, Garcia JR, Miller GT, Satin AJ, Baschat AA. Ultrasound-based three-dimensional printed medical model for multispecialty team surgical rehearsal prior to fetoscopic myelomeningocele repair. Ultrasound in Obstetrics & Gynecology. 2018;**51**(6):836-837

[60] Chen SA, Ong CS, Hibino N, Baschat AA, Garcia JR, Miller JL. 3D printing of fetal heart using 3D ultrasound imaging data. Ultrasound in Obstetrics & Gynecology. 2018;**52**(6):808-809

[61] DeVore GR, Klas B, Satou G, Sklansky M. 24-segment sphericity index: A new technique to evaluate fetal cardiac diastolic shape. Ultrasound in Obstetrics & Gynecology. 2018;**51**(5):650-658

[62] DeVore GR, Satou G, Sklansky M. Abnormal fetal findings associated with a global sphericity index of the 4-chamber view below the 5th centile. Journal of Ultrasound in Medicine. 2017;**36**(11):2309-2318

[63] Hobbins JC, Gumina DL, Zaretsky MV, Driver C, Wilcox A, DeVore GR. Size and shape of the four-chamber view of the fetal heart in fetuses with an estimated fetal weight less than the tenth centile. American Journal of Obstetrics and Gynecology. 2019;**221**(5):495-4e1

[64] Hamet P, Tremblay J. Artificial intelligence in medicine. Metabolism. 2017;**69**:S36-S40

[65] Yasutomi S, Arakaki T, Matsuoka R, Sakai A, Komatsu R, Shozu K, et al. Shadow estimation for ultrasound images using auto-encoding structures and synthetic shadows. Applied Sciences. 2021;**11**(3):1127

[66] LeCun Y, Bengio Y, Hinton G. Deep learning. Nature. 2015;**521**(7553):436-444

[67] McDonald M, Salisbury H. Physical activity, exercise, and musculoskeletal disorders in sonographers. Journal of Diagnostic Medical Sonography. 2019;**35**(4):305-315. DOI: 10.1177/8756479319843883

[68] Park J, Sofka M, Lee S, Kim D, Zhou SK. Automatic nuchal translucency measurement from ultrasonography. In: Medical Image Computing and Computer-Assisted Intervention–MICCAI 2013: 16th International Conference, Nagoya, Japan, September 22-26, 2013, Proceedings, Part III 16 2013. Berlin Heidelberg: Springer; 2013. pp. 243-250

[69] Pluym ID, Afshar Y, Holliman K, Kwan L, Bolagani A, Mok T, et al. Accuracy of automated three-dimensional ultrasound imaging technique for fetal head biometry. Ultrasound in Obstetrics & Gynecology. 2021;**57**(5):798-803

[70] Yeo L, Romero R. New and advanced features of fetal intelligent navigation echocardiography (FINE) or 5D heart. The Journal of Maternal-Fetal & Neonatal Medicine. 2022;**35**(8):1498-1516

[71] Ferrier C, Dhombres F, Khoshnood B, Randrianaivo H, Perthus I, Guilbaut L, et al. Trends in resource use and effectiveness of ultrasound detection of fetal structural anomalies in France: A multiple registry-based study. BMJ Open. 2019;**9**(2):e025482

[72] Carrera JM, Torrents M, Mortera C, Cusi V, Munoz A. Routine prenatal ultrasound screening for fetal abnormalities: 22 years' experience. Ultrasound in Obstetrics and Gynecology: The Official Journal of the International Society of Ultrasound in Obstetrics and Gynecology. 1995;**5**(3):174-179

[73] Ubavić M, Durković M, Kis T. Prenatal screening markers for down syndrome: Sensitivity, specificity, positive and negative expected value method. Journal of Medical Biochemistry. 2018;**37**(1):62

Chapter 4

Perspective Chapter: Next-Generation Sequencing and Variant Cataloging for Screening and Diagnosis of Sphingolipidoses and Mucopolysaccharidoses

Irina Vlasova-St. Louis, Uri Barak and Svetlana Khaiboullina

Abstract

This chapter provides a comprehensive examination of how next-generation sequencing (NGS) technologies are transforming prenatal and neonatal care, particularly in the diagnosis of lysosomal diseases (LDs). These rare, inherited conditions are caused by defects in lysosomal metabolism. If not detected and treated early, they can lead to significant disabilities and reduced life expectancy. The chapter specifically focuses on the use of NGS to diagnose and screen sphingolipidoses (SLDs) and mucopolysaccharidoses (MPSs). It covers the molecular pathogenesis, classification, and main symptomatology of the diseases. The chapter reviews the progress made in identifying the genes associated with SLDs and MPSs and cataloging clinically relevant genetic variants. Additionally, it highlights the growing adoption of NGS for diagnosis and screening by institutions such as academic research centers, private healthcare providers, and government health agencies. It also discusses the challenges in NGS implementation, regulation, and outlines future directions for its application in prenatal and neonatal medicine.

Keywords: lysosomal diseases (LDs), sphingolipidoses (SLDs), mucopolysaccharidoses (MPSs), next-generation sequencing (NGS), whole exome sequencing (WES), whole genome sequencing (WGS), genetic variant classification and curation, variant pathogenicity, phenotype/genotype correlation, newborn screening, carrier screening

1. Introduction

In modern medical diagnostics, genetic testing plays a critical role in identifying hereditary conditions that, if undetected during the first few days or months of life, can lead to severe disabilities or significantly reduce life expectancy.

Among the most transformative applications of genetic testing is its use in peri-neonatal diagnostics and screening, particularly through next-generation sequencing (NGS). This cutting-edge technology has revolutionized prenatal and neonatal diagnosis, enabling early detection of genetic disorders and effective disease prevention through carrier screening [1]. NGS technologies, including whole exome sequencing (WES), whole genome sequencing (WGS), and targeted panel sequencing, have become integral tools in clinical laboratories for uncovering genetic variants. These techniques are particularly valuable in neonatal intensive care units (NICUs), where they facilitate the diagnosis of rare genetic diseases, congenital anomalies, and metabolic disorders that are often undetectable using conventional methods [2]. By offering unparalleled sensitivity and specificity, NGS not only accelerates the diagnosis of genetic conditions but also informs personalized treatment protocols and improves prognosis [3]. Additionally, its capability to detect ultra-rare or previously unde-scribed genetic disorders underscores its significance in advancing medical research.

Inborn errors of metabolism (IEM) constitute a large proportion of the conditions screened during the neonatal period [4]. IEM-underlying disorders are characterized by a wide range of symptoms and complications, making them difficult to diagnose using traditional approaches. NGS-based newborn screening offers a comprehensive solution by identifying genetic variations associated with IEM. This early detection enables healthcare providers to implement personalized management strategies, optimizing long-term health outcomes for affected newborns [5]. Furthermore, the ability of NGS to detect a broad spectrum of rare and novel metabolic conditions highlights its superiority over conventional biochemical screening methods [6].

The importance of addressing metabolic disorders is reflected in international classification efforts. The International Classification of Diseases 11th Revision (ICD-11) now includes a broader range of IEMs, signifying their increasing relevance in global health [7]. The presence of "unspecified" (Z) and "other specified" (Y) categories in ICD-11's classification of metabolic diseases reflects the ongoing challenges in definitively categorizing these complex disorders. The extension .0Z serves as a provisional classification for unclear diagnoses, while .0Y accommodates rare variants and newly discovered conditions that do not align with established classifications. This hierarchical system highlights both the rapid evolution of our understanding and the current limitations in creating distinct categories for every known variant, particularly affecting ultra-rare conditions and atypical presentations. This classification system enables standardized diagnosis and improved clinical management across healthcare system. Complementing this effort, the International Classification of Inherited Metabolic Disorders (ICIMD) provides a detailed categorization of biochemical pathways, with a particular focus on lysosomal metabolism disorders (commonly referred to as lysosomal diseases). These pathways are vital for the breakdown and recycling of intracellular molecules [8].

Building on this foundation, this chapter explores the use of NGS as a diagnostic and screening tool for lysosomal diseases (LDs). It highlights recent advancements by academic medical centers, private hospitals, and governmental organizations in identifying and cataloging clinically relevant genetic variants. The focus is placed on two major groups of LDs - sphingolipidoses and mucopolysaccharidoses - discussing advances in classification, challenges in implementation, and future directions for integrating NGS into clinical and public health laboratories.

2. Lysosomal diseases (LDs, ICD-11code: 5C56.0Y, 5C56.0Z)

Lysosomal diseases (formerly, lysosomal storage diseases) encompass a diverse group that recently exceeded seventy inherited disorders affecting lysosomal metabolism due to defects in enzymes, transporters, or other proteins essential to lysosomal function. Although each individual LDs are rare, conjointly they represent a significant number of cases worldwide, ranging up to 23 per 100,000 live births [9]. Most LDs follow an autosomal recessive inheritance pattern [10]. This means that an affected child is born to phenotypically healthy parents, who are heterozygous for the genetic variants (carry one copy of the mutated gene) and are unaware of their carrier status. As a result, families may lose a child to the disease or endure a lengthy diagnostic odyssey before a diagnosis is made.

The molecular mechanisms underlying LDs, along with the genetic backgrounds of affected individuals, display considerable variability, leading to a wide spectrum of clinical symptoms and presentations [10]. Currently, the combination of genetic and biochemical tests has proven to increase success of the diagnostic utility.

2.1 Diagnostic challenges

Biochemical tests, while valuable for diagnosis of LDs, present challenges in harmonizing testing procedures and minimizing false positive and false negative results [11]. Typically, these tests detect metabolic byproducts in urine, plasma, or dried blood spots, often employing tandem mass spectrometry assay (described in introductory chapter) [12]. There are numerous (laboratory-developed) biochemical assays that directly measure the activity of affected enzymes [11]. However, they are difficult to multiplex, making them labor-intensive and time-consuming. Additionally, there is limited biochemical correlation between enzyme levels in dried blood spots and actual disease phenotypes [13]. This complicates interpretation of test results and assessment of the prognosis [14]. Premature newborns, in particular, have a significantly higher rate of results that fall into gray area and requiring the test to be repeated [15]. This increases the cost and period of diagnostic uncertainty for families.

2.2 Opportunity for NGS

NGS-based tests offer the potential for earlier and more accurate diagnosis, even in premature babies. In clinical settings, many companies, such as Prevention Genetics (now part of Exact Sciences) offer custom panels that include 10 to 242 genes implicated in lysosome-related disorders. The panels for newborn screening are also in the development: for example, the NEOseq_ACTION panel has tested 254 genes designed to diagnose neonates with LDs and other metabolic conditions [16]. Although newborn sequencing for LDs is primarily conducted in clinical settings, several public health laboratories in the United States and other countries have incorporated targeted NGS into newborn screening programs for conditions such as Mucopolysaccharidosis types I and II, Krabbe disease, and Pompe disease [17, 18].

NGS is instrumental for diagnosis of unexplained developmental delays, organomegaly, and neurological deterioration, associated with unknown hereditary metabolic conditions [19–21]. However, a key challenge for NGS lies in accurately assessing gene-disease associations and determining the pathogenicity of genetic variants (also referred to here as mutations) [22]. The analysis of NGS as a diagnostic or screening procedure presents challenges in assigning variant classification and identifying putative disease-causing mutations. As of today, a large proportion of variants is classified as variants of uncertain significance (VUS). Additionally, conventional NGS protocols have limited detection of the complex rearrangements and large indels (except for KaryoSeq HD) [23]. To address these limitations, orthogonal techniques such as array-based comparative genomic hybridization (aCGH), a multiplex ligation-dependent probe amplification (MLPA), a polymerase chain reaction-restriction fragment length polymorphism (PCR-RFLP), or cDNA analysis by Sanger sequencing, must be employed to complement the NGS molecular analysis. Predicting the late onset of LDs through mutational analysis remains challenging, especially in the absence of neonatal symptoms [24]. Currently, neither NGS nor biochemical tests alone can accurately predict the late onset forms or assess the milder forms of the disease. As a result, both technologies will likely continue to be used in the future to delineate LDs pathology, correlate phenotypes, and predict disease progression [25].

3. Identification and classification of mutations in affected LDs genes

LDs are caused by a wide range of genetic mutations that impair lysosomal function. These mutations disrupt various biochemical pathways within lysosomes, which are essential for the degradation and recycling of cellular waste [26]. NGS, introduced over a decade ago, has been a breakthrough tool for diagnosing LDs, helping families end their diagnostic odyssey [27]. Nevertheless, predicting phenotypic effect and onset and course of the disease for novel combinations of pathogenic variants, particularly those in a compound heterozygous state, remains challenging. The genotype-phenotype relationship in LDs is complex. Individuals who are homozygous for pathogenic variants in LD-causing genes develop severe forms of the respective disorders characterized by early onset and rapid progression. In contrast, other types of mutations, such as missense mutations, may lead to milder forms of the disease, with later onset and slower progression. The severity often depends on the specific mutation and whether the individual has compound heterozygosity (two or more different mutations in the same gene).

This chapter includes links to ClinVar and the Human Gene Mutation Database (HGMD) databases in **Table 1**, highlighting genes and mutations that cause specific lysosomal diseases (SLDs and MPSs). The ClinVar database is a part of the US National Center for Biotechnology Information (NCBI) organization. It compiles genetic variants of clinically relevant genes and populated by approved volunteer-submitters. The HGMD is owned and curated by Qiagen Inc., and it also catalogs gene variants associated with genetic disorders, including LDs. These databases are practical resources for researchers and clinicians, who assess the pathogenicity of genetic variants following the standards, developed by American College of Medical Genetics and Genomics (ACMG) and Association for Molecular Pathology (AMP) [28]. ACMG's 2015 standards for sequence variant interpretation are world-wide accepted guidelines to classify genetic variants according to five main categories. In brief, this classification combines genetics with clinical, familial, populational, functional, and computational evidence for pathogenicity [28].

Various types of mutations reported in LDs. The most clinically significant are nonsense, frameshift, gross insertions/deletions/duplications or other complex rearrangements, as well as splicing mutations that result in exon skipping, or intron retention. In cases where clinical data is lacking, the pathogenicity of missense variants associated with LDs is often assessed using computational programs that predict (*in silico*) the variant's impact on protein structure and function [29]. Variants predicted to be harmful are more likely to be disease-causing and to contribute to the development of the condition, particularly when backed by evidence such as functional studies and significant differences in their frequency between affected individuals and the general

Disease	Affected Gene	Chr	Total	P	LP	VUS	Conflict	B/LB	Web link
Sphingolipidoses									
GLD	GALK	14q31	1434	248	198	326	73	446	https://www.ncbi.nlm.nih.gov/clinvar/?term=GALC%5Bgene%5D&redir=gene https://www.hgmd.cf.ac.uk/ac/gene.php?gene=GALC
GD	GBA1	1q21	359	106	87	124	40	42	https://www.ncbi.nlm.nih.gov/clinvar/?term=GBA https://www.hgmd.cf.ac.uk/ac/gene.php?gene=GBA
Fabry	GLA	Xq22	1234	489	188	295	82	250	https://www.ncbi.nlm.nih.gov/clinvar/?term=GLA%5Bgene%5D&redir=gene https://www.hgmd.cf.ac.uk/ac/gene.php?gene=GLA
Farber	ASAH1	8p22-p21.3	1005	133	61	343	27	459	https://www.ncbi.nlm.nih.gov/clinvar/?term=ASAH1%5Bgene%5D&redir=gene https://www.hgmd.cf.ac.uk/ac/gene.php?gene=ASAH1
MLD	ARSA	22q13.31-qter	1298	343	170	317	57	459	https://www.ncbi.nlm.nih.gov/clinvar/?term=ARSA%5Bgene%5D&redir=gene https://www.hgmd.cf.ac.uk/ac/gene.php?gene=ARSA
CPSAPD	PSAP	10q21-q22	922	65	33	250	63	543	https://www.ncbi.nlm.nih.gov/clinvar/?term=PSAP%5Bgene%5D https://www.hgmd.cf.ac.uk/ac/gene.php?gene=PSAP
GM1	HEXA	15q23-q24	1160	196	144	354	37	488	https://www.ncbi.nlm.nih.gov/clinvar/?term=hexa%5Bgene%5D&redir=gene https://www.hgmd.cf.ac.uk/ac/gene.php?gene=HEXA
GM2	HEXB	5q13	817	137	90	175	30	414	https://www.ncbi.nlm.nih.gov/clinvar/?term=HEXB%5Bgene%5D&redir=gene https://www.hgmd.cf.ac.uk/ac/gene.php?gene=HEXB
GM3	ST3GAL5	2p11.2	477	51	14	196	17	206	https://www.ncbi.nlm.nih.gov/clinvar/?term=ST3GAL5%5Bgene%5D&redir=gene https://www.hgmd.cf.ac.uk/ac/gene.php?gene=ST3GAL5
GM2AB	GM2A	5q31.3-q33.1	227	18	7	108	1	95	https://www.ncbi.nlm.nih.gov/clinvar/?term=GM2A%5Bgene%5D&redir=gene https://www.hgmd.cf.ac.uk/ac/gene.php?gene=GM2A

Disease	Affected Gene	Chr	Total	P	LP	VUS	Conflict	B/LB	Web link
NPD A/B	SMPD1	11p15.4-p15.1	1039	207	204	178	112	414	https://www.ncbi.nlm.nih.gov/clinvar/?term=SMPD1%5Bgene%5D&redir=gene https://www.hgmd.cf.ac.uk/ac/gene.php?gene=SMPD1
NPD C1	NPC1	18q11-q12	2498	375	306	554	174	1237	https://www.ncbi.nlm.nih.gov/clinvar/?term=NPC1%5Bgene%5D&redir=gene https://www.hgmd.cf.ac.uk/ac/gene.php?gene=NPC1
NPD C2	NPC2	14q24.3	285	41	34	61	15	154	https://www.ncbi.nlm.nih.gov/clinvar/?term=NPC2%5Bgene%5D&redir=gene https://www.hgmd.cf.ac.uk/ac/gene.php?gene=NPC2
Mucopolysaccharidoses									
MPSI	IDUA	4p16.3	2156	347	159	672	94	986	https://www.ncbi nlm.nih.gov/clinvar/?term=IDUA%5Bgene%5D&redir=gene https://www.hgmd.cf.ac.uk/ac/gene.php?gene=IDUA
MPSII	IDS	Xq28	1581	749	302	173	53	491	https://www.ncbi.nlm.nih.gov/clinvar/?term=IDS%5Bgene%5D&redir=gene https://www.hgmd.cf.ac.uk/ac/gene.php?gene=IDS
MPS IIIA	SGSH	17q25.3	1480	130	112	536	76	696	https://www.ncbi.nlm.nih.gov/clinvar/?term=SGSH%5Bgene%5D&redir=gene https://www.hgmd.cf.ac.uk/ac/gene.php?gene=SGSH
MPS IIIB	NAGLU	17q21	1276	170	132	406	57	559	https://www.ncbi.nlm.nih.gov/clinvar/?term=NAGLU%5Bgene%5D https://www.hgmd.cf.ac.uk/ac/gene.php?gene=NAGLU
MPS IIIC	HGSNAT	8p11.1	1258	144	71	402	40	630	https://www.ncbi.nlm.nih.gov/clinvar/?term=hgsnat%5Bgene%5D&redir=gene https://www.hgmd.cf.ac.uk/ac/gene.php?gene=HGSNAT
MPS IIID	GNS	12q14	761	64	19	232	15	440	https://www.ncbi.nlm.nih.gov/clinvar/?term=GNS%5Bgene%5D&redir=gene https://www.hgmd.cf.ac.uk/ac/gene.php?gene=GNS

DOI: http://dx.doi.org/10.5772/intechopen.1009417

Disease	Affected Gene	Chr	Total	P	LP	VUS	Conflict	B/LB	Web link
MPS IVA	GALNS	16q24.3	1378	245	178	355	124	546	https://www.ncbi.nlm.nih.gov/clinvar/?term=GALNS%5Bgene%5D https://www.hgmd.cf.ac.uk/ac/gene.php?gene=GALNS
MPS IVB	GLB1	3p21.33	1170	193	150	261	57	569	https://www.ncbi.nlm.nih.gov/clinvar/?term=GLB1%5Bgene%5D&redir=gene https://www.hgmd.cf.ac.uk/ac/gene.php?gene=GLB1
MPS VI	ARSB	5q11-q13	967	156	156	267	42	400	https://www.ncbi.nlm.nih.gov/clinvar/?term=ARSB%5Bgene%5D&redir=gene https://www.hgmd.cf.ac.uk/ac/gene.php?gene=ARSB
MPS VII	GUSB	7q21.11	668	72	33	192	24	359	https://www.ncbi.nlm.nih.gov/clinvar/?term=GUSB%5Bgene%5D&redir=gene https://www.hgmd.cf.ac.uk/ac/gene.php?gene=GUSB
MPS IX	HYAL1	3p21.3- p21.2	376	46	2	118	11	204	https://www.ncbi.nlm.nih.gov/clinvar/?term=HYAL1%5Bgene%5D&redir=gene https://www.hgmd.cf.ac.uk/ac/gene.php?gene=HYAL1

Chr, chromosomal location. P, pathogenic variants; LP, likely pathogenic; VUS, variants of uncertain significance; B, Benign; LB, likely benign Conflicting, conflicting classifications, submitted by various clinical genetic providers.
Note: This data was accessed between Aug-Sept 2024. HGMD access is granted with basic account subscription (free account establishment is required). The instructions on how to navigate ClinVar and HGMD can be found here:
https://www.ncbi.nlm.nih.gov/clinvar/docs/help/.
https://www.youtube.com/watch?v=D-Rd036FbXM.

Table 1.
Genes implicated in lysosomal diseases with chromosomal position (extracted from HGMD) and the number of classified gene variants (extracted from ClinVar).

population [30, 31]. Many remain classified as variants of uncertain significance (VUS) due to their rarity and limited evidence, which is common in rare diseases like LDs where small patient cohorts hinder clear pathogenic links. More research and clinical data are needed to understand the significance of these VUS and their role in LDs. In this chapter, we provide multiple examples of genes with pathogenic variants linked to disorders of glycosphingolipid and glycosaminoglycan degradation.

4. Disorders of glycosphingolipid degradation

4.1 Genes affected in sphingolipidoses (ICD-11 codes: 5C56.0Z, 5C56.0Y)

Sphingolipidoses (SLDs) comprise a diverse group of genetic disorders characterized by the accumulation of sphingolipids within cells and tissues due to deficiencies in specific lysosomal enzymes required for their degradation [32]. The buildup of sphingolipids, such as sphingomyelin, glucocerebroside, or ceramide, can lead to dysfunction and damage in multiple organs throughout the body. The specific symptoms and severity of sphingolipidoses vary depending on the type of sphingolipid that accumulates in the affected organs [33].

The sphingolipid degradation pathway is complex, with SLDs biochemically categorized into primary and secondary types [34, 35]. Primary SLDs result from enzyme deficiencies directly within the sphingolipid degradation pathway [35, 36]. In contrast, secondary SLDs arise from deficiencies in other proteins that affect glycosphingolipid catabolism indirectly [36, 37]. Recently developed liquid chromatography coupled with tandem mass spectrometry-based test (LC-MS/MS) multiplexed detections of four biomarkers of SLDs [37]. Because early diagnosis and intervention are crucial for managing the progression of these disorders, the implementation of NGS in neonatal screening has significant medical utility in improving patient outcomes.

4.2 Pathogenic variants in the GALC gene are causative for globoid cell leukodystrophy (GLD) (ICD-11 code: 8A44.4)

Mutations in the GALC gene result in the deficiency of the enzyme galactosylceramidase (also known as galactocerebrosidase), which underlays the pathology of globoid cell leukodystrophy (also Krabbe disease) (**Table 1**) [38]. This enzyme is essential for the hydrolysis of galactolipids, particularly in the central nervous system and kidneys [38]. The inability to break down galactolipids results in the accumulation of toxic substances, leading to the progressive neurological deterioration seen in GLD [39]. Traditionally, Globoid Cell Leukodystrophy is screened through biochemical methods, such as measuring enzyme activity and the biomarker psychosine [38]. However, these methods can sometimes yield false positive results, underscoring the need for molecular diagnostic confirmation. This is particularly important in the infantile form of Krabbe disease, which is a deadly condition requiring urgent intervention in newborn period [40–42]. Early treatment, such as a hematopoietic stem cell transplantation, is most effective if performed before 30 days of life [43]. The inclusion of infantile Krabbe disease in the Recommended Uniform Screening Panel (RUSP) in 2024 by Public Health Programs in the USA marks a significant public health advancement [44]. This milestone enables the future implementation of next-generation sequencing (NGS) as a screening method in newborn screening programs, potentially facilitating earlier diagnosis and timely interventions to improve outcomes.

Pathogenic variants in GALC have been extensively studied. Loss-of-function mutations (null variants), or those resulting in significant protein truncation, are responsible for the severe infantile form of GLD [45–47]. Certain combinations of missense variants may cause late infantile onset [48]. Adult onset of Krabbe is usually caused by missense variants (e.g., p.L634S) or whole exon deletions [46, 49, 50]. Adult onset Krabbe can present as an accidental finding on MRI imaging along with general clinical findings such as seizures, spastic paraplegia, or sudden onset of cognitive decline [49–51]. Moreover, mutations in GALC have been implicated in conditions with dual rare genetic diseases, such as the co-occurrence of Angelman syndrome and Krabbe disease [52].

Krabbe disease is economically burdensome due to the costs associated with treatment and long-term care. By using NGS for carrier screening, healthcare providers can identify individuals with heterozygous GALC mutations. This proactive approach allows for early intervention and informed family planning, which can significantly reduce the long-term costs of managing the disease [53]. Genetic counseling further supports this strategy by helping families understand their risk and make informed decisions, thereby mitigating the financial and emotional impact of Krabbe disease.

4.3 Pathogenic variants in the GBA1 are causative for glucocerebrosidosis types 1–3 (Gaucher disease, GD)

Gaucher disease (glucocerebrosidosis types 1–3) is the most common form of LDs. It is caused by pathogenic variants in glucosylceramidase beta 1 (GBA1) gene that encodes the acid β-glucosidase (also known as glucocerebroside, GCase) enzyme [54]. GCase catalyzes the conversion of glucosylceramide (GlcCer) into ceramide and glucose. The deficiency/absence of this enzyme leads to the accumulation of glycolipid glucocerebroside (glucosylceramide), primarily in the spleen, liver, and bone marrow, affecting cellular signaling and function [55]. There are different types of GD, such as type 1 (non-neuronopathic), type 2 (acute neuronopathic), and type 3 (chronic neuronopathic), which vary in severity and the presence or absence of neurological symptoms [56, 57]. Several public health laboratories in the USA and rare disease centers worldwide have implemented newborn screening programs for Gaucher disease. After initial positive screening results, patients are referred to specialized clinics for comprehensive biochemical monitoring. This monitoring extends beyond basic GCase enzyme assessment to include multiple biomarkers such as glycosylsphingosine (lyso-Gb1) and glycosylsphingosine chitotriosidase 1 (CHIT1), which can be measured in both blood and cerebrospinal fluid [56, 58–60]. However, the reliability of biochemical monitoring remains challenging, as these tests frequently yield false positive or false negative results. Such diagnostic uncertainty complicates clinical decision-making processes and may lead to misinterpretation of disease status, highlighting the need for improved diagnostic strategies [61].

NGS has become a commonly used diagnostic tool for GD. Several studies attempted to differentiate GD types, based on patient's genetics [62]. The assessment of the GBA1 gene faces challenges due to the presence of pseudogene. It should be noted that it is located close to a pseudogene called GBAP1, which is a non-functional copy of the GBA1 gene [63]. The presence of the glucosylceramidase beta pseudogene 1 (GBAP1), which is highly homologous to the functional GBA1 gene, complicates genetic testing using NGS technologies [64]. The pseudogene and the functional gene share significant sequence similarity, making it challenging to distinguish between mutations in the functional gene and pseudogene [65]. Additionally, recombinations between two genes, complicate identification and location of the specific mutations responsible for GD [66]. Therefore, MLPA verification, as well as careful molecular analysis to parse mutations in GBA1 from GBAP is required [67, 68]. Recently, long-read NGS was used to sequence GBA1 and adjacent regions to identify individuals, carrying a recombinant allele [69]. According to research results, long-read NGS did not outperform pair-end short-read NGS, and still required orthologous confirmatory assay [69]. Thus, many clinical investigators prefer to order GBA1 PCR–RFLP, or Sanger dideoxy sequencing for patients suspected of having GD [62, 70, 71].

The genotype-phenotype relationship in Gaucher disease has been extensively studied. It was shown that the common variant p.L483P is associated with GD types 2–3, while p.N409S mutation was found in GD type 1 [72]. Despite these findings, significant challenges remain in predicting the future disease course, particularly in infants. For this reason, continuous reassessment of variant classifications, as well as close monitoring of patients, is crucial to ensure accurate prognosis and appropriate medical intervention. This helps address the variability in clinical outcomes that can arise, even among individuals with the same mutations [73–75].

In recent years, there has been a significant advances in our understanding of GBA1 variants (as outlined in **Table 1**). The International Working Group on Gaucher Disease (IWGGD) has proposed standardized diagnostic procedures to improve consistency in GD management [76]. However, progress in establishing a robust genotype-phenotype relationship has been hampered by challenges such as inconsistent data sharing and limitations in DNA banking within GD registry platforms [77].

With the availability of ERT for Gaucher disease, which provides partial therapeutic effect, the importance of early diagnosis has grown. NGS, especially in newborn screening NGS, is now believed to be timely. The early diagnosis can help address critical issues like neurological dysfunction and prevent severe complications such as skeletal abnormalities and cytopenia [78]. Moreover, the link between glucocerebrosidase gene mutation carrier status and the increased genetic risk for developing Parkinson's disease emphasizes the importance of NGS-based carrier screening as a precision diagnostic test for making informed reproductive decisions [79].

4.4 Pathogenic variants in the GLA gene are causative for Fabry disease (FD) (ICD-11 code: 5C56.01)

FD is an X-linked lysosomal disease caused by a mutation in a gene called galactosidase A gene (GLA), leading to a deficiency of the enzyme α-galactosidase A (AGAL). Enzyme deficiency leads to the accumulation of globotriaosylceramide (Gb3) primarily affecting the kidneys, heart, and nervous system [80]. In hemizygous males, Fabry disease generally presents in two forms: classic form, with symptoms usually beginning in childhood or adolescence (e.g., corneal opacity, acroparesthesia, angiokeratomas, hypohidrosis) [81]. Symptoms may appear later in adulthood (late-onset form) and are usually associated with common pathogenic variant p.R112H (**Table 1**) [82].

Historically, heterozygous females were considered as asymptomatic carriers of X-linked disorders, as the presence of one normal X chromosome was thought to be sufficient to prevent the full expression of the disorder [83]. However, recent findings have shown that females can exhibit a wide range of clinical symptoms, including atypical presentations of FD with renal and cardiac pathology [84, 85]. Therefore, it is important to diagnose not only affected male newborns but also female carriers.

To date, almost 1300 variants have been described, with 446 of them being pathogenic or likely pathogenic, and nearly the same number of VUS (**Table 1**) [86]. There were cases where familial FD was initially diagnosed based on biochemical test results. Later identified genetic variants that were previously classified as benign in older literature, were reclassified based on new evidence [87, 88]. Various ERTs are available to help mitigate myocardial fibrosis and renal complications in Fabry disease, underscoring the importance of NGS in precision diagnosis [89, 90].

4.5 Pathogenic variants in the ASAH1 are causative for Farber's lipogranulomatosis (FRBRL) and related disorders

FRBRL is a disease linked to a deficiency in the enzyme acid ceramidase (ACD), which is encoded by the ASAH1 gene (N-acylsphingosine amidohydrolase) (**Table 1**). Pathogenic variants in ASAH1 can result in two extremely rare genetic disorders: FRBRL and Spinal Muscular Atrophy with Progressive Myoclonic Epilepsy (SMA-PME) [91]. Recent research suggests that these two disorders may represent a spectrum of acid ceramidase deficiency conditions rather than entirely separate diseases [92, 93]. The NGS and detailed variant analysis are crucial in identifying disease-causing genetic variants for ASAH1-related disorders, including well known, such as p.R153C and p.G307S [94]. There are more reports about novel mutations in ASAH1 for SMA-PME (including p.P37T and p.T42M) [95–98].

FRBRL is classified as sphingolipidosis, although its molecular pathogenesis is not well understood. Traditionally, FRBRL was divided into 4 types, based on the age of onset:

- Classic, with symptoms appearing between 2 weeks to 4 months of age;
- Intermediate, which typically begins around 9 months of age;
- Mild disease, with symptoms emerging between 2 to 20 months of age;
- Neonatal visceral disease, where symptoms such as hepatosplenomegaly are present at birth due to massive histiocyte infiltration of organs like the liver and spleen, as well as the lungs, thymus, and lymph nodes [92, 99, 100].

The classic, intermediate, and mild forms of the disease often have symptoms of subcutaneous nodules, laryngeal abnormalities, painful joint contractures, and neuromuscular impairment [91]. In addition to molecular testing and NGS, histological analysis of tissue biopsies typically reveals granulomatous infiltration, foam cells, and lysosomes with characteristic comma-shaped, curvilinear tubular structures known as Farber's bodies [101].

The body of knowledge surrounding the genetics of FRBRL/SMA-PME and ASAH1 mutations' spectrum is continually expanding (**Table 1**) [102]. Functional studies of pathogenic variants, identified in cases of fetal demise, provided the insights into molecular pathogenesis, particularly highlighting the abnormal splicing caused by the c.458-2A > T mutation [103]. Additionally, mutational analyses using mouse models and functional studies in patient leukocytes have played a key role in clarifying why symptoms may vary among patients [98, 104]. As research advances, these disorders are likely to undergo reclassification. A deeper understanding of the genetic variants within the ASAH1 gene, alongside their biochemical mechanisms, may lead to their organization into a unified category. This category would accurately reflect the shared enzyme deficiency responsible for these conditions, helping to streamline diagnoses and inform treatment approaches.

4.6 Pathogenic variants in the ARSA gene are causative for metachromatic leukodystrophy (MLD) (ICD-11 code: 5C56.02)

MLD is a sphingolipidosis that is characterized by the inability to degrade sulfatides, mainly the galactosyl-3-sulfate ceramides. It is caused by deficient activity of lysosomal enzyme arylsulfatase A, due to pathogenic single nucleotide variants (SNV) in the arylsulfatase A (ARSA gene) [105, 106]. This enzyme deficiency results in the accumulation of sulfatides (specifically cerebroside sulfate) within the lysosomes of oligodendrocytes and Schwann cells, leading to the progressive demyelination characteristic of MLD [107].

Patients can present symptoms in late infantile, juvenile, or adult age, which include psychomotor and cognitive decline (with various degrees of progression), seizures, and eventually, paralysis [108, 109]. Adult onset of MLD is often misdiagnosed as multiple sclerosis or other neurodegenerative and psychiatric diseases [110, 111]. It was noted that a spectrum of compound heterozygous mutations persists in consanguineous communities from various countries and regions of the world [112–114]. Rare variants identified by WGS include not only missense, but also in-frame duplications, and the pathogenic variants in other leukodystrophies genes (e.g., SUMF1, PSAP) [115–117].

Genetic testing for ARSA is now part of most NGS panels for diagnosing LDs, facilitating early diagnosis, and even presymptomatic screening of newborns as per recent consensus guidelines [118–120]. The algorithms, predicting the disease severity are under development, though they are not yet fully established [118]. While there is no cure for MLD, allogeneic stem cell transplantation is used as a treatment option to slow disease progression [121]. Given the genetic basis of the disease, genetic counseling for families with affected children and NGS carrier screening of relatives are essential strategies for preventing of the disease in future generations [122, 123].

4.7 Pathogenic variants in the PSAP gene are causative for combined PSAP deficiency (CPSAPD)

CPSAPD is an ultra-orphan condition. All types of mutations, including deletions, insertions, splice site mutations, and missense mutations, were reported in PSAP (**Table 1**). The PSAP gene encodes prosaposin mRNA, which is processed and translated into four saposin proteins: A, B, C, and D [124]. A deficiency in these proteins disrupts the degradation of sphingolipids, leading to the pathological accumulation of these lipids within lysosomes, particularly affecting neurons [125].

CPSAPD has a complex phenotype that reflects the essential roles of saposins in sphingolipid metabolism. The disease is often misdiagnosed with atypical Gaucher, Krabbe, and other glycosphingolipid degradation disorders [126, 127]. The polymorphism in the PSAP gene is also linked to Parkinson's disease [128, 129].

Given the intricate genetic factors underlying CPSAPD pathology and the frequent involvement of multiple genes (e.g., ARSA [117]), prioritizing NGS for differential diagnosis, as well as carrier screening for informed family planning and genetic risk assessment, is crucial.

4.8 Genes affected in GM1, GM2 and GM3 gangliosidoses

Gangliosidoses are considered a subset of sphingolipidoses. Gangliosides are a specific type of sialic acid-containing sphingolipids with localization in neuronal membranes [130]. Gangliosidoses are characterized by excessive accumulation of specific gangliosides in the central nervous system [131]. Neurodegeneration usually progresses rapidly, resulting in a poor prognosis with patients rarely surviving into adulthood [132]. NGS testing can be used to identify mutations in the relevant genes, confirming the diagnosis of gangliosidoses and providing information about the specific subtype. Preconception genetic risk assessment is crucial for GM genetic counseling, as there is no cure for these disorders. The treatment is supportive (focusing on managing symptoms), or experimental and under investigation [133, 134].

4.8.1 Pathogenic variants in the GLB1 gene are causative for GM1 gangliosidosis

GM1 gangliosidosis is caused by mutations in the GLB1 gene, which encodes the enzyme β-galactosidase. Mutations in the same gene are also responsible for mucopolysaccharidosis type IV (see subchapter 5.4.2). The deficiency in β-galactosidase leads to the accumulation of GM1 gangliosides (GM1G) in neurons, contributing to skeletal dysostosis and neurodegenerative symptoms of the disorder [135]. There are three subtypes of GM1 gangliosidosis based on the age of onset and severity: infantile, late infantile, and juvenile/adult forms [135, 136].

Variations in the nature and location of mutations within the GLB1 gene (as listed in **Table 1**) account for differences in the loss of enzyme activity. Location of these mutations within the gene's functional domains directly impacts the enzyme β-galactosidase's ability to degrade GM1G, leading to various levels of disease severity [137]. Mutations that disrupt regions essential for substrate processing typically result in more severe disease phenotypes (e.g., p.R201C, p.W273L, p.I51T). In contrast, mutations in less critical regions may cause milder forms of the disease (e.g., p.R457Q, p.T500A, p.N462K) [137, 138]. This variability in mutations explains the range of clinical manifestations observed in GM1 gangliosidosis.

Based on Next-Generation Sequencing (NGS) data and our understanding of GLB1 gene mutations, individualized gene therapy treatments are currently being tested in clinical trials NCT03952637 and NCT04713475. These trials are investigating the efficacy and safety of personalized gene therapies aimed to correct specific genetic defects in patients with GM1 gangliosidosis, utilizing gene transfer techniques to restore the function of the defective GLB1 gene [133].

Additionally, single nucleotide polymorphisms (SNP) in the GLB1 gene have been associated with other neurological disorders, including Alzheimer's, Parkinson's, and Huntington's disease [138].

4.8.2 Genes affected in GM2 gangliosidoses

Two proteins are affected in GM2: 1. β-hexosaminidase A which is composed of one α-subunit (encoded by HEXA gene) and one β-subunit (encoded by HEXB gene), and 2. β-hexosaminidase B, consisting of two β-subunits (encoded by HEXB).

4.9 Pathogenic variants in the HEXA gene cause Tay-Sachs disease (TSD) (ICD-11 code: 5C56.00)

Mutations in the HEXA gene lead to a deficiency or complete absence of the HEX A enzyme (the α-subunit of β-hexosaminidase A). These mutations result in the accumulation of GM2 gangliosides within the neurons of the brain and spinal cord [139]. Progressive neurodegeneration, cherry-red spots in the macula, and persistent strabismus are hallmarks of TSD [140]. The onset, symptoms, and rate of progression depend on total hexosaminidase activity as well as functional and structural imbalance between HEX subunits (HEX A and HEX B) [141, 142].

TSD is more commonly seen in people who are of Ashkenazi Jewish or French-Canadian descent (males and females are equally affected) [143]. The frequency of pseudodeficiency may also be higher in these populations, thus representing a diagnostic conundrum estimating whether the proband is truly affected and what would be the expected onset of the disease [139]. A number of well-reported pathogenic variants with clinical cases are cataloged in HGMD and ClinVar (**Table 1**) (e.g., p.R499C, p.R504H, p.R504C, p.M1T, p.Q106*, c.1073 + 1G > A, c.571-1G > T, etc.) [140, 144, 145].

The molecular pathology of TSD is complex, however, key mechanisms can be outlined as: 1) defects of enzyme folding, preventing it from adopting the correct conformation necessary for its function; 2) defects in enzyme chains assembly or misfolding that can disrupt the assembly process; 3) trafficking defects: misfolded proteins may be recognized by the cell's quality control systems and targeted for degradation before they can reach the lysosome [146].

Prenatal and preconception genetic screening, as well as the screening populations at risk, are of utmost importance for TSD since there is still no cure for this deadly condition [147].

4.10 Pathogenic variants in the HEXB contribute to GM2 gangliosidosis (Sandhoff disease)

The Sandhoff disease caused by mutations in the HEXB gene that encode a β-subunit of β-hexosaminidase. In Sandhoff disease, both β-hexosaminidase A (which consists of α- and β-subunits) and β-hexosaminidase B (made of two β-subunits) enzymes are defective [148]. These mutations cause the accumulation of GM2 gangliosides and globosides in various tissues [149].

Newly discovered variants identified by NGS (e.g., homozygous frameshift p.A40fs*24 or gross deletion g.74012742_74052694del) have been reported in single case studies (**Table 1**) [150, 151]. Since the hexosaminidase A enzyme (described above) is composed of one α-subunit and one β-subunit, the mutations in the HEXB gene also lead to reduced or absent HEX A enzyme activity. Thus, both HEX A and HEX B activities, as well as the total hexosaminidase activity, are decreased depending on the severity of the mutations in the HEXB gene [152, 153]. The presence of pathogenic variants in other genes (e.g., MYH7) could complicate the clinical presentation and lead to overlapping or additional symptoms that are not solely attributed to Sandhoff disease [154]. This presents challenges in diagnosis, as variant classifications in either HEX gene alone cannot serve as the sole basis for clinical judgment. It requires the use of specific algorithms that incorporate both biochemical and genetic studies [155].

4.11 Pathogenic variants in the GM2A gene contribute to GM2 gangliosidosis AB variant

The GM2A gene encodes for the GM2 ganglioside activator protein (GM2A, also GM2AP) (**Table 1**). This protein plays a crucial role in the metabolism of GM2 gangliosides, acting as a substrate-specific cofactor for β-hexosaminidase A. The β-hexosaminidase hydrolyses GM2 gangliosides releasing GM3 gangliosides [137, 156]. GM2AP binds to GM2 gangliosides and presents them to HEX A, for degradation within the lysosomes [157].

GM2 gangliosidosis AB has about thirty documented cases in the literature with the combination of variants reported being p.K27* and p.P139S [158]. Patients with GM2 activator deficiency exhibit symptoms of neurodegeneration, similar to TSD and Sandhoff diseases (typically presenting in early childhood), because this genetic defect affects the same metabolic pathway [138, 159]. Thus, biochemical analysis of HEX enzyme activities alone is not sufficient to diagnose GM2 AB [160–162]. Information on GM2 AB can also be found through the National Tay-Sachs and Allied Diseases Association websites (NTSAD).

4.11.1 Pathogenic variants in the ST3GAL5 gene cause GM3 gangliosidosis

Pathogenic variants in the ST3GAL5 gene (ST3 β-galactoside α-2,3-sialyltransferase 5) cause sialyltransferase enzyme deficiency and GM3 gangliosidosis [163]. This enzyme adds sialic acid to glycoproteins and glycolipids, which is essential for the synthesis of GM3 gangliosides [164]. Loss of sialyltransferase function results in the accumulation of gangliosides (sphingolipids with sialic acid) in neurons, leading to developmental regression, intellectual disability, motor dysfunction, seizure, and choreoathetosis [165–167]. The most common pathogenic variant identified in the French, Pakistani, African American, and North American Amish populations, is p.R288Ter [163, 168]. As observed in other genetic conditions, the location of pathogenic variants can greatly impact the level of residual enzyme activity [165, 169].

An alternative clinical form of GM3 gangliosidosis is the salt and pepper developmental regression syndrome (SPDRS), which presents with distinctive clinical symptoms [170]. The SPDRS is characterized by salt-and-pepper-like appearance of skin dyspigmentation along with progressive neurological decline [171]. Both conditions share a genetic cause but seem to differ in the mutational spectrum and their clinical presentation and progression [170, 172]. Future re-classification may group both conditions under a common name GM3 synthase deficiency (GM3SD) or ST3GAL5-related conditions, reflecting their shared biochemical basis [163].

4.12 Genes affected in sphingomyelinase deficiencies

Sphingomyelinases are a specific subset of sphingolipidoses that involve the abnormal metabolism and accumulation of sphingomyelin due to acid sphingomyelinase enzyme deficiency (ASMD), also known as Niemann-Pick disease types A, B, and C [173, 174].

4.12.1 Pathogenic variants in the SMPD1 gene are affected Niemann-Pick disease type A and B (NPA and NPB)

NPA and NPB are caused by mutations in the sphingomyelin phosphodiesterase 1 (SMPD1) gene, leading to a decreased activity of lysosomal acid sphingomyelinase (ASM) [175]. The enzyme ASM is mainly present in lysosomes, where it hydrolyzes the sphingomyelin (SM) to ceramide and phosphocholine. Different types of pathogenic variants for NPA and NPB were described in the literature, with mutations ranging from missense to small and large indels [176–180].

The genetic nature of mutations for ASMD type A is more severe (e.g., nonsense and frameshifts which are classified as "pathogenic very strong" according to ACMG standards) [181, 182]. Clinical symptoms of NPA include an early onset of disease (infantile), neurological involvement, muscular atrophy, and developmental delay [178, 179, 183]. Laboratory findings in the bone marrow usually show lipid-laden foamy histiocytes in the bone marrow and macular cherry-red spots on the fundoscopic exam [179, 184].

In contrast, NPB usually manifests later in life with symptoms such as hepatosplenomegaly (and occasionally adrenal enlargement) and abnormal hematological findings [185]. The most common SMPD1 variant associated with NPB is p.R610del [177, 186]. Many novel variants related to NPB have been discovered through NGS during differential diagnosis of unexplained hepatosplenomegaly [187–189]. Although combined mutations in SMPD1 and other genes are extremely rare, a few cases have been reported, such as mutations in the tyrosine hydroxylase gene, highlighting the significance of WES or WGS for accurate diagnosis [188, 190]. It is particularly important to rule out acid sphingomyelinase deficiency in patients with suspected glucosylceramidase beta deficiency (Gaucher disease). Both conditions can present with similar clinical symptoms, such as hepatosplenomegaly and other organ pathologies, making accurate diagnosis essential for proper management [191, 192]. NGS carrier screening is becoming more popular in countries where the prevalence of NPD A/B is high [186].

The introduction of recombinant human ASM (olipudase alfa, Xenpozyme®) in 2022 is a significant advancement in treatment of ASMD, particularly type B, which primarily presents with non-central nervous system manifestations [193]. Olipudase alfa has been shown to reduce ASMD mortality and morbidity over a two-year treatment period, underscoring the critical importance of early genetic diagnosis [194]. The global regulatory approval of this biologic agent has led to updates in disease management guidelines and recommendations for monitoring this phenotypically and genotypically complex condition [192, 195].

4.12.2 Pathogenic variants in the NPC1 and NPC2 cause Niemann-Pick disease type C

Mutations in the NPC1 or NPC2 genes disrupt the intracellular transport of cholesterol and lipid within cells, leading to the pathological accumulation of these substances and resulting in the clinical manifestations of Niemann-Pick disease type C (NPC) [196]. These proteins (NPC intracellular cholesterol transporter 1 Niemann-Pick type C1 and C2) function together in the membranes of late endosomes and lysosomes [197]. NPC1 and 2 are essential for moving cholesterol out of lysosomes [198]. The disease is typically characterized by a progressive neurodegenerative course with symptoms that can include ataxia, vertical supranuclear gaze palsy, psychosis, dystonia, respiratory distress, hepatosplenomegaly, and in severe cases, neonatal death [199–204].

Approximately 2500 variants in the NPC1 gene have been documented, whereas fewer (285) have been reported in the NPC2 gene in databases such as ClinVar and HGMD (**Table 1**). This discrepancy could be related to a recent GWAS study indicating reduced fertility in heterozygotes for NPC2 mutations [205]. Lower fertility rates could lead to fewer carriers of NPC2 mutations, thereby decreasing the chance of two carriers having offspring with NPC. The diverse mutations in NPC1 and NPC2 genes result in a broad spectrum of phenotypic presentations [180, 206–211]. The detection of NPC1 or NPC2 mutations is frequently an incidental finding during NGS panel workups for diagnosis of other LDs [212, 213]. Therefore, it is important to test both NPC1 and NPC2 genes for a conclusive genetic diagnosis [214]. Identifying novel mutations, and assessing genetic variants for pathogenicity based on the ACMG standards would strengthen the clinical utility of genetic testing and empower informed genetic counseling of affected individuals and their families [206].

Currently, there is no cure for NPC, and treatment remains symptomatic and supportive. Miglustat is a drug that inhibits ganglioside synthesis and has shown effectiveness in slowing the progression of neurological symptoms [215]. This drug is also approved for use in Gaucher disease [216]. On August 2, 2024, the FDA genetic metabolic diseases advisory committee (GeMDAC) voted favorably for the approval of the investigational drug arimoclomol for NPC treatment [217]. For more information about NPC and updates on experimental treatments, readers are encouraged to visit the Hide and Seek Foundation for Lysosomal Disease Research and the Niemann-Pick Disease Foundation (NNPDF) websites.

In summary, sphingolipidoses are rare monogenic diseases typically diagnosed at specialized medical centers. However, there is growing support from medical experts, non-profit organization, like National Organization for Rare Disorders (NORD), and patient advocacy groups to include these metabolic disorders in recommended newborn screening panels.

5. Disorders of glycosaminoglycan metabolism

5.1 Genes affected in mucopolysaccharidoses (MPSs) (ICD-11 code: 5C56.3)

MPSs are a group of LDs caused by deficiencies in lysosomal enzymes responsible for the degradation of glycosaminoglycans (GAGs). These disorders result in accumulation of GAGs (including keratan sulfate and chondroitin-6-sulfate), in various tissues throughout the body, leading to progressive multiorgan dysfunction and a wide range of clinical manifestations (**Figure 1**) [218]. The clinical manifestations of MPSs vary widely, ranging from severe infantile-onset forms with rapid progression to milder forms with symptoms appearing later in life [219, 220]. The severity and presentation of MPSs depend on the specific enzyme deficiency, the degree of enzyme activity, and the amount and distribution of accumulated GAGs [220]. GAGs are long sugar chains vital for the structure and function of tissues such as cartilage, skin, and the extracellular matrix [218].

There are 11 recognized subtypes of MPSs, each associated with deficiencies in specific lysosomal enzymes and characterized by distinct clinical features (**Figure 1**). All MPSs are considered rare, with estimated incidences ranging from 1 to 7 per 100,000 live births depending on the country [221, 222].

While several common founder mutations have been identified in certain populations for some MPS types, the phenomenon of pseudodeficiency complicates diagnosis. Pseudodeficiency refers to genetic variants that reduce enzyme activity but do not cause clinical symptoms of MPS [223]. These variants can confound diagnostic testing and lead to false-positive results [223]. Therefore, biochemical assessment of GAG levels and enzyme activity is instrumental for confirming the diagnosis of MPS and distinguishing between true enzyme deficiencies and pseudodeficiency.

Brusius-Facchin et al. assessed the sensitivity and specificity of the NGS panel for detecting genetic mutations in patients with MPSs who had been previously diagnosed and genotyped by Sanger sequencing [224]. The NGS method identified

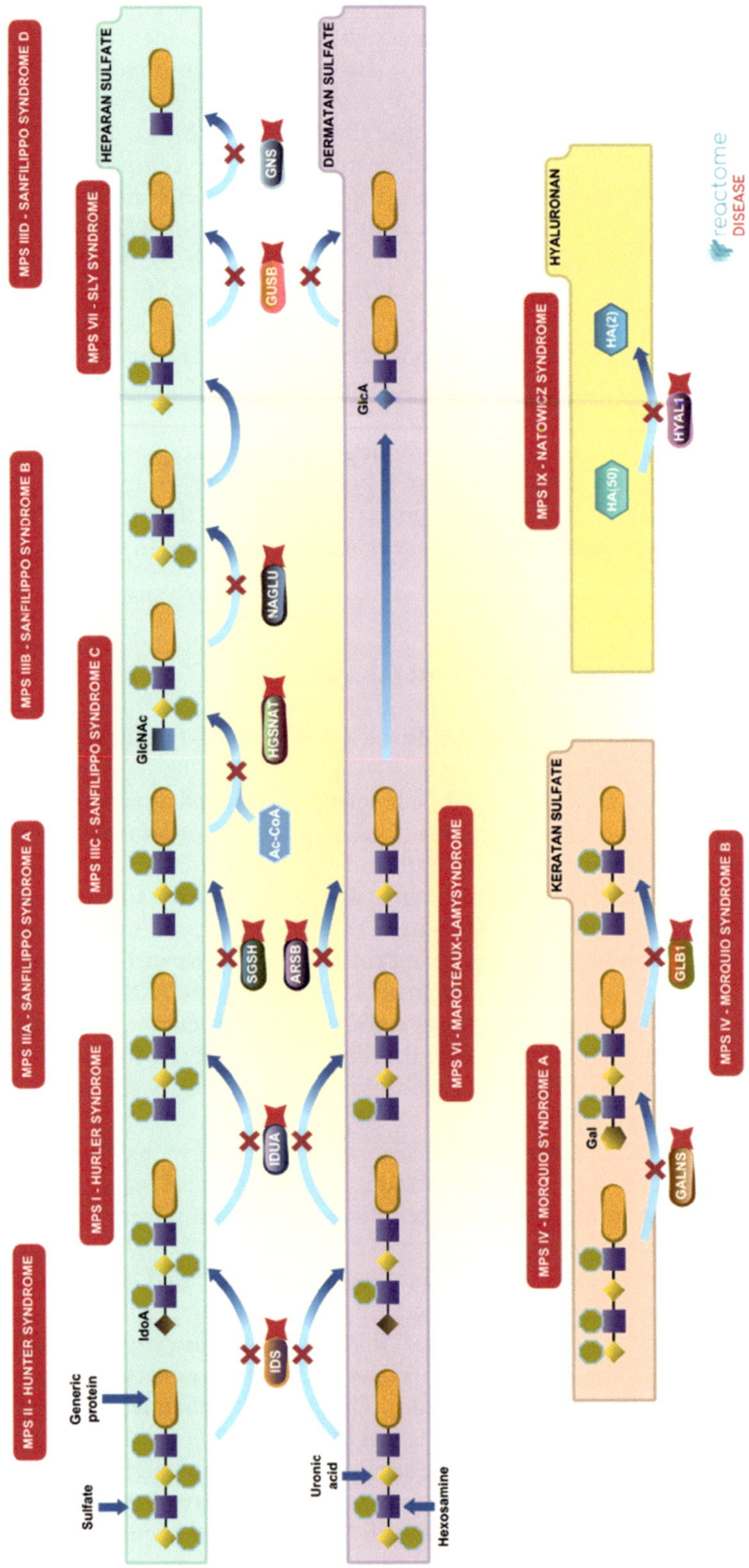

Figure 1.
There are 11 known enzyme deficiencies that give rise to 7 distinct MPS types. This pathway is available at Reactome.org https://reactome.org/PathwayBrowser/#/R-HSA-2206281.

96% of the variants previously found with Sanger sequencing, confirming its high sensitivity, while no new variants were detected, ensuring 100% specificity, suggesting NGS is suitable as the first-tier assay [224]. By implementing a two-tier diagnostic approach, workflow can be optimized: NGS can serve as the first tier screening tool, identifying potential genetic mutations associated with MPSs, followed by biochemical confirmation as the second-tier to validate the findings and provide a definitive diagnosis. This approach enhances the accuracy and efficiency of MPS diagnoses, which is important for timely intervention and management [224].

5.2 Pathogenic variants in the α-L-iduronidase (IDUA) gene are causative for MPS I

Pathogenic variants in the IDUA gene are implicated in Mucopolysaccharidosis type I (MPS I, ICD-11 code: 5C56.30), an autosomal recessive lysosomal disorder [225]. The IDUA gene encodes the enzyme α-L-iduronidase, which is essential for breaking down glycosaminoglycans (GAGs), specifically dermatan sulfate and heparan sulfate (**Figure 1**).

MPS I was historically classified into three subtypes - Scheie, Hurler-Scheie, and Hurler syndromes - based on the age of onset and severity of symptoms. MPS I exhibits a spectrum of phenotypes ranging from severe (classical) to intermediate and attenuated forms due to a wide range of α-L-iduronidase deficiencies [226, 227]. The disease involves multiorgan pathology and manifests with symptoms like coarse facies, valvular heart disease, corneal clouding, hepatomegaly, kyphosis gibbus, dysostosis multiplex, pigmentary retinopathy, and cognitive impairment, among others [228]. If left undiagnosed and untreated, MPS I can lead to fatal outcomes in infancy, underscoring the importance of public health initiatives that incorporate testing for IDUA enzyme deficiency using heel-prick dried blood spot screening methods [226]. In recognition of this need, MPS I disease was added to the USA Recommended Uniform Screening Panel (RUSP) in 2016.

A number of pathogenic variants have been identified and submitted to ClinVar, with 347 classified as pathogenic, 159 as likely pathogenic, and 672 as variants of uncertain significance (**Table 1**). Notable IDUA variants are presented in NCBI GeneReviews and peer-reviewed publications [229]. Different pathogenic variants in the IDUA gene confer various phenotypic manifestations of MPS I, with some variants leading to more severe disease manifestation than others [230, 231]. Homozygous missense mutations (p.A327P, p.W402C, p.R89Q, p.Q70E, p.G51D) that abrogate IDUA's catalytic domain, as well as pathogenic truncating variants (p.Q70X, p.W402X) are typically associated with the severe and early onset of MPS I [232–235]. This form of the disease requires hematopoietic stem cell transplantation for treatment [236]. There are over a hundred variants that contribute to an intermediate severity phenotype or late disease onset when present in compound heterozygosity [237]. The combination of variants with different levels of pathogenicity presents a diagnostic challenge [238]. A recent report described a biallelic genotype of nonsense and missense variants that produced an attenuated MPS I phenotype of a 38-year-old patient [239].

NGS is now considered a standard test, enabling early diagnosis and management of MPS I in many countries [31, 240, 241]. Several public health institutions are utilizing dried blood spots for detecting pathogenic mutations in the IDUA gene as a second-tier test [240–244]. However, the presence of pseudodeficiencies in the IDUA gene poses significant challenges in screening healthy newborns using NGS [245].

Combining biochemical data with NGS results helps to identify and catalog pseudodeficiency variants, which are typically associated with a modest reduction in IDUA enzyme activity and normal urine GAG levels [244, 246]. Several studies have identified pseudodeficiency variants, such as p.A79T and p.H82Q, as compound heterozygous with VUS or with each other [246, 247]. This co-occurrence leads to diagnostic uncertainty and necessitates patient follow-ups and continuous biochemical monitoring of urine GAGs throughout childhood [246]. Pseudodeficiency can also complicate treatment decisions. MPS I is currently managed using enzyme replacement therapy (ERT), which involves weekly infusions of laronidase and can only be prescribed to those with a definitive diagnosis [248].

The accumulated genetic and phenotypic evidence from patient registries will enhance the diagnosis of MPS I based on reported genotype-phenotype relationships. In 2018, ClinGen (Clinical Genome Resource at NIH) established the first Lysosomal Diseases Variant Expert Panel (VCEP), which specifically focuses on IDUA gene variant classifications and submissions to ClinVar. This committee developed a variant classification standard operating procedure specifically tailored for analyzing variants in the IDUA gene.

5.3 Pathogenic variants in the iduronate 2-sulfatase gene (IDS) are causative for MPS II (Hunter syndrome)

Mucopolysaccharidosis type II (MPS II, ICD-11 code: 5C56.31), also known as Hunter syndrome, differs from MPS I in its genetic basis and mode of inheritance [249]. In MPS II, the affected gene is iduronate 2-sulfatase (I2S). The pathogenic variants are transmitted via an X-linked recessive inheritance pattern [250]. MPS II symptoms are largely overlapped with other MPSs and include developmental delay, behavioral problems, coarse facial features, enlarged organs, hearing and vision loss, and joint stiffness, which makes differential diagnosis near impossible without knowing the genetic cause [227].

To date, 749 pathogenic variants, 302 likely pathogenic variants, and 173 VUS have been reported to ClinVar (**Table 1**). However, very few of these mutations are associated with early-onset forms of the disorder [251]. The attenuated forms of MPS II appear to be more common but are not detectable by biochemical methods at birth [251, 252]. Most missense mutations in the IDS gene are associated with the attenuated form, which is characterized by a later onset of symptoms [253]. Recombination between the IDS gene and its pseudogene IDS2 can be detected via NGS, but confirmatory tests are required for validation and ongoing monitoring of late-onset cases [254].

Severe MPS II cases often involve frameshift deletions, such as c.1270delG, and whole exon deletions [224, 255]. RNA-sequencing analysis can validate rare splice-junction defects and IDS-EOLA1 gene fusions, as reported in [256]. In an extremely rare case of Hunter syndrome in a female child reported by Semyachkina et al., a structural defect affecting the Xq28 region resulted in a hemizygous state for a mutation inherited from the mother [257].

A recent study demonstrated that NGS is a more effective method than Sanger sequencing for detecting mosaic events in carrier mothers of MPS II patients, providing greater sensitivity and accuracy [258]. Unlike Sanger sequencing, which provides a cumulative signal, NGS analyzes individual DNA read, making it easier to detect low level mosaicism in mothers, which is important for genetic counseling and estimation of the recurrence risk of transmitting the same mutation to male and female offsprings [258].

In summary, while clinical genetic laboratories can now accurately diagnose MPS II, predicting genotype-phenotype correlation remains a challenge [240]. Early diagnosis through genetic testing is highly advantageous, as demonstrated by the effectiveness of early treatment with the FDA-approved ERT drug idursulfase for severe forms of MPS II [259]. Given the benefits of presymptomatic treatment, the US Secretary of Health and Human Services added MPS II to the RUSP in August 2022 [260].

5.4 Genes affected in mucopolysaccharidosis type III

MPS III is perhaps the most phenotypically and genotypically diverse type of MPSs. It is divided into four subtypes based on the affected genes, with each subtype having its unique biochemical and clinical features, depending upon the level of intracellular accumulation of heparan sulfate [220]. Despite these differences, all subtypes share common symptoms such as progressive neurodegeneration (including retinal degeneration), developmental delay, intellectual disability, behavioral problems, sleep disorders, and skeletal abnormalities [261–263]. The severity and age of onset of symptoms can vary widely among affected individuals, even within the same subtype, contributing to the observed phenotypic and genotypic diversity in MPS III [261, 264]. Novel pathogenic and pseudodeficiency alleles are reported regularly in the literature and databases like HGMD or ClinVar (**Table 1**) [265]. Although there are ongoing pharmacological research efforts to test novel therapeutics for MPS III, no treatments have been approved yet. Currently, most patients do not survive beyond adolescence, underscoring the importance of carrier screening and early diagnosis through NGS [266, 267].

5.4.1 Pathogenic variants in the SGSH are causative for MPS IIIA (Sanfilippo type A)

Mutations in the N-sulfoglucosamine sulfohydrolase (SGSH) gene underlie the pathology of MPS IIIA (ICD-11 code: 5C56.32). A total of 242 clinically significant mutations (classified as pathogenic/likely pathogenic variants) are listed for the SGSH gene in ClinVar (**Table 1**). Interpretation of these variants can be challenging, particularly in the absence of clear disease phenotypes [268–270]. Although biochemical tests are valuable for diagnosis of MPS IIIA, they have challenges such as the limited availability of enzyme testing (in blood leukocytes or fibroblasts), which is typically offered only in centralized laboratories performing NGS [271].

Collecting and storing comprehensive clinical data, including genotype-phenotype correlations, treatment outcomes, and disease progression, is also challenging [222]. Without robust data collection and storage mechanisms, accurately correlating specific SGSH gene mutations with the clinical manifestations of MPS IIIA remains difficult [270].

5.4.2 Pathogenic variants in the NAGLU are causative for MPS IIIB (Sanfilippo type B)

Mutations in the NAGLU gene, which encodes α-N-acetylglucosaminidase, result in MPS IIIB disorder. A total of 1276 variants have been reported in the NAGLU gene in ClinVar (**Table 1**), of which 170 are classified as pathogenic and 132 as likely pathogenic. Various compound heterozygous mutations have been documented (e.g., p.W168Ter/p.M1?) [272]. Certain mutations are associated with earlier onset or more severe symptoms, while others may lead to milder or atypical forms of the disease [273–275]. Severe forms of the disease are often linked to consanguinity within families, making segregation analysis valuable for identifying carriers in extended family members [276]. Several case reports describe the co-inheritance of mutations in NAGLU and other genes like CYP26B1 or GCDH, which were detected by WES [277, 278]. This underscores the importance of WES in diagnosis of MPS IIIB and rare diseases in general. As our understanding of NAGLU mutations grows and genetic test interpretations become more refined, clinicians may be able to diagnose MPS IIIB shortly after birth, allowing for early intervention and management [279].

5.4.3 Pathogenic variants in the HGSNAT are causative for MPS IIIC (Sanfilippo type C)

The HGSNAT gene encodes heparan-α-glucosaminide N-acetyltransferase. Mutations in this gene are responsible for MPS IIIC (**Table 1**). Sanfilippo type C is characterized by early-onset progressive neuronal demyelination caused by accumulation of intracellular heparan sulfate [280, 281]. ClinVar has documented submissions for 1258 mutations in the HGSNAT gene, including pathogenic, likely pathogenic, and variants of uncertain significance (VUS) (see **Table 1**). The largest proportion of pathogenic mutations are a missense variants; however, recent NGS studies identified numerous splice variants, frameshifts and small pathogenic deletions [265, 282–284]. Additionally, mutations in the HGSNAT gene are associated with late onset nonsyndromic retinitis pigmentosa (RP) [285–287]. Several RP-specific alleles have recently been reported, that are different from those identified in MPS IIIC [282, 283, 288, 289].

As more individuals undergo genetic testing for MPS IIIC, the accuracy of variant classification is expected to improve. Asymptomatic individuals can be identified through carrier screening. Early identification of carriers can benefit the genetic counseling when planning a family, especially in regions with high rates of consanguinity [265, 284].

5.4.4 Pathogenic variants in the GNS are causative for MPS IIID (Sanfilippo type D)

MPS IIID is an ultra-rare disease characterized by the accumulation of partially degraded heparan sulfates in lysosomes, leading to cellular damage, particularly affecting neurons [290]. There are few well-described variants in the GNS gene (N-acetylglucosamine-6-sulfatase) that cause the MPS IIID disease, as recorded in ClinVar (**Table 1**) [265, 291]. These variants often cluster within specific families [291, 292]. Currently, there is no treatment for MPS IIID, but preclinical studies have shown some promise for ERT using recombinant human α-N-acetylglucosamine-6-sulfatase in a mouse model [293]. The development of biochemical newborn screening test for MPS IIID is currently in progress [294]. In the meantime, NGS may play a crucial role in empowering family planning through GNS carrier screening analysis.

5.5 Genes affected in MPS IVA, MPS IVB, MPS VI, MPS VII, and MPS IX. (ICD-11 code: 5C56.3Y)

Like MPS I, these MPS subtypes are also inherited in an autosomal recessive fashion [265]. Cases of these MPS subtypes tend to co-segregate within families and share similar clinical profiles and phenotypes, with occasional multigenic nature [295]. Symptoms of MPSs IV-IX are similar and include skeletal abnormalities, joint laxity, short stature, corneal clouding, organomegaly, and potentially life-threatening complications affecting the respiratory and cardiovascular systems [265].

Biochemical tests are unable to differentiate between these MPS subtypes due to the similar accumulation of partially degraded GAGs within lysosomes (e.g., hyaluronan, chondroitin-, keratan-, or dermatan- sulfates) [295]. Knowledge about variant pathogenicity for these forms of MPSs is limited. Therefore, sequencing of the patient and parents (trio sequencing) is the only way to identify causative pathogenic variants, particularly those in a compound heterozygous state.

5.5.1 Pathogenic variants in the GALNS are causative for MPS IVA (Morquio A)

The mutational spectrum of the galactosamine-6-sulfatase (GALNS) gene, associated with MPS IVA (Morquio syndrome type A, ICD-11 code: 5C56.32), is broad (see **Table 1**). Mutations in the GALNS gene lead to a dysfunction or loss of activity of the GALNS enzyme, which results in severe or attenuated phenotypes [296]. With the rapid implementation of NGS in clinical laboratories, numerous mutations have been identified in patients worldwide [297–299]. Certain mutations in the GALNS gene have been recorded at higher frequencies than others, suggesting the possibility of founder effects [298, 300]. Very rarely, the second pathogenic variant may not be detected through standard DNA sequencing [301]. In such cases, next-generation mRNA sequencing can be used to identify multiple splicing RNA isoforms, particularly when mutations are located in deep intronic regions that affect splicing [301]. In fact, the deep intronic variant c.128_138delGCGATGCTGAG (p.Gly43Aspfs*5) was identified as common in the mild form of MPS IVA [299]. Dual gene mutations (e.g., GALNS and BTD, Biotinidase) have been reported to present with a combination of symptoms from both conditions and demonstrate a strong segregation component [265]. Studies employing both mutational and segregation analyses contribute to our understanding of the molecular basis of MPS IVA [302]. Also, collected data could help uncover the complex interplay between genetic variation, population history, and variation in disease phenotype [299]. Early diagnosis and access to ERT treatment is imperative to maintain quality of life for these patients.

5.5.2 Pathogenic variants in the GLB1 are causative for MPS IVB (Morquio B disease) and GM1 gangliosidosis

Mutations in the GLB1 gene lead to the development of MPS IVB and/or GM1 gangliosidosis [303]. GLB1 encodes β-galactosidase, which plays a role not only in degradation of GAGs but also gangliosides and oligosaccharides [304–306]. The dual pathology arises from a deficiency of the β-D-galactosidase enzyme, resulting in the accumulation of ganglioside GM1 and keratan sulfates [307, 308]. A key clinical distinction of MPS IVB (and IVA) is that cognitive function is typically unaffected, unlike MPS types like MPS I, II, or III, where neurological symptoms are common. When keratan sulfate accumulation is dominant, patients are diagnosed with MPS IVB, which is characterized by pronounced dysostosis multiplex [309, 310].

Few well-described variants in GLB1 have been reported (18 likely pathogenic and 64 pathogenic, **Table 1**) as associated with both MPS IVB and GM1 [304]. One of the most common mutations associated with MPS IVB is the p.W273L, frequently found among European MPS IVB patients [303, 305]. Additionally, variants like p.T500A and p.R201H have only been detected in patients with MPS IVB, suggesting the existence of genotype-phenotype correlations [222]. Therefore, considering biochemical results and prioritizing screening for clinically relevant variants, can help differentiate MPS IVB from GM1 [222, 304, 307].

5.5.3 Pathogenic variants in the ARSB mutations are the genetic cause of MPS VI (Maroteaux-Lamy syndrome)

MPS VI is also known as Maroteaux-Lamy syndrome (ICD-11 code: 5C56.33). It is caused by mutations in the ARSB gene that lead to a deficiency or malfunctioning of the arylsulfatase B enzyme, which is involved in the breakdown of GAG dermatan sulfate [311]. Like MPS IV, individuals with MPS VI generally have normal intelligence, but have short stature and more prominent skeletal deformities.

The data on ARSB variants in ClinVar and HGMD is very limited (**Table 1**). In some segregations, certain mutations in the ARSB gene are more prevalent, many of which are missense, nonsense, or small deletions [31, 271, 311–315]. Mutations in ARSB translational start site and deep intronic regions were reported to cause the disease, highlighting the importance of WGS in improving the diagnostic rate of these rare disease-causing variants [316, 317]. The most common alleles are p.L321P (in the Turkish population) and p.Y251* (in the Arabic population) [318]. Diagnosis typically involves NGS panel testing, along with measuring GAG levels in urine and the activity of the arylsulfatase B enzyme in blood or fibroblasts [319]. However, early diagnosis is important for managing symptoms with the ERT drug galsulfase, marketed under the brand name Naglazyme [319].

5.5.4 Pathogenic variants in the GUSB are causative for MPS VII (Sly syndrome)

MPS VII, also known as Sly syndrome, is a very rare disease caused by mutations in the GUSB gene, which encodes the enzyme β-glucuronidase [320]. This enzyme plays a crucial role in processing GAGs, such as dermatan sulfate and heparan sulfate [321]. The onset of symptoms is documented in infancy or later in childhood, and the severity of MPS VII can range from mild to life-threatening (hydrops fetalis), depending on the degree of enzyme deficiency [321].

The mutational spectrum of the GUSB gene associated with MPS VII is diverse (**Table 1**). A various types of mutations are identified, linking to the most severe form of MPS VII such as prenatal nonimmune hydrops fetalis and fetal demise (e.g., homozygous p.R36L, or p.A442T) [322, 323]. The musculoskeletal, neurological, sensory, cardiac, and respiratory features of MPS VII are similar to the other MPSs [324–328].

102 pathogenic mutations were described in the GUSB gene (see **Table 1**), including missense/nonsense mutations, splicing mutations, regulatory mutations involving CpG islands, as well as small deletions and gross deletions [321, 329, 330]. The spectrum and frequency of these mutations can vary based on the geographic and ethnic background of the patients' population. The missense p.L176F was reported as the most frequent worldwide [331, 332]. Pseudodeficiency alleles and *de novo* mutations have also been described [26, 323].

Identifying and sharing pathogenic GUSB variants is important due to the life-threatening nature of MPS VII [333]. Prenatal and newborn NGS testing is recommended for affected families, as it could facilitate the early treatment with recombinant vestronidase alfa, which has demonstrated effectiveness in phase 3 clinical trials [333, 334].

5.5.5 Pathogenic variants in the HYAL1 are causative for MPS IX (Natowicz syndrome)

MPS IX is caused by mutations in the hyaluronoglucosaminidase 1 gene (HYAL1), which is involved in the breakdown of hyaluronic acid [335]. Information on mutations in MPS IX is limited due to an extremely rare nature of the disease (**Table 1**). MPS IX is often diagnosed in the context of familial juvenile idiopathic arthritis [88].
Genetic testing is crucial for confirming a diagnosis of MPS IX, especially in cases where clinical manifestations are ambiguous or overlap with other conditions.
Understanding the genetic basis of MPS IX and identifying specific mutations, in the HYAL1 gene, are essential for accurate diagnosis, genetic counseling, and potential future therapeutic interventions for affected individuals and their families.

In conclusion, significant progress has been made in understanding the genetic mechanisms underlying MPS disorders. Clinical genetic laboratories rely on expert variant curators to evaluate and classify the pathogenicity of novel variants based on ACMG guidelines and FDA-recognized classification frameworks [336]. The classification of MPS disorders continues to evolve. While labels like MPS V and MPS VIII have been retired and are no longer associated with any conditions, most MPS disorders are now considered clinically actionable. This indicates that identifying genetic variants associated with these diseases enables early clinical intervention, effective management strategies, or informed decision-making, which can improve the patient's health outcomes. Furthermore, new types of MPS are expected to be identified, supported by findings from animal models (e.g., ARSK deficiency-related MPS [337], or VPS33A gene-related MPS-plus syndrome [338]). These conditions are anticipated to be described in humans as NGS becomes increasingly accessible [337]. More information can be found on the National MPS Society (UK) and Hunter's Hope Foundation websites.

6. Precision genetics, future perspectives

The gene-to-disease approach for diagnosing genetic conditions, including LDs, is gaining popularity due to its cost-effectiveness and potential to improve patients' quality of life [339]. WES and WGS are increasingly ordered by physicians as diagnostic and screening tools because they can identify genetic variations linked to nearly 10,000 rare inherited conditions (see Orpha.net website) [340]. NGS tests for SLDs and MPSs, offered by private genetic services as part of LD or carrier screening panels, provide comprehensive genetic insights for affected individuals and their families. In addition to enhancing diagnostic capabilities, these panels support personalized management strategies [18, 341].

To facilitate the widespread use of NGS panels, WES and WGS for diagnosis of germline diseases, cross-laboratory standardization is essential for both NGS techniques and variant pathogenicity interpretation [342, 343]. In 2024, the FDA published its final ruling on the oversight of Laboratory Developed Tests (LDTs), including NGS tests, marking a significant shift in regulatory policy [344]. This new framework will be implemented over a five-year period, divided into five stages [345]:

"Stage 1 (Effective 05/2025): Laboratories must comply with requirements for medical device reporting, correction and removal reporting, and complaint file management.

Stage 2 (Effective 05/2026): New requirements for establishment registration, device listing, labeling, and investigational use of LDTs will be enforced.

Stage 3 (Effective 05/2027): Laboratories must implement a compliant quality system, including auditing, design controls, and risk management.

Stage 4 (Effective 10/2027): Premarket review requirements for high-risk (Class III) IVDs offered as LDTs must be met.

Stage 5 (Effective 05/2028): Premarket review requirements for moderate- and low-risk IVDs offered as LDTs must be met."

The FDA will continue to allow some discretion in enforcement, particularly for NGS-LDTs used in integrated healthcare systems or those approved by New York State's Clinical Laboratory Evaluation Program (CLEP). This flexibility will help laboratories transition smoothly to the new regulatory framework without disrupting patient care [345, 346].

New regulatory requirements also underscore the need for uniformly reporting actionable genetic variants, differentiating between clinically significant (deleterious) variants and potentially relevant variants like VUS. As mentioned above, germline variant interpretation is currently guided by the ACMG and AMP [28]. The expanding ClinGen projects aim to build and support a robust infrastructure for interpreting genetic variants within the context of human health and disease [347]. Within ClinGen, Clinical Domain Working Groups (CDWGs) focus on specific areas of clinical genetics, such as cardiovascular diseases, hereditary cancers, and inborn errors of metabolism, including lysosomal disease gene curation panels [347, 348].

The systematic collection and storage of genetic and clinical data are crucial for understanding genetic disease progression and informing treatment strategies. One such initiative is the Genome Connect patient registry, integrated into ClinGen, which encourages affected families to share de-identified data with laboratories. This data-sharing effort helps refine variant classification and promotes collaboration among laboratories to resolve conflicting interpretations in ClinVar, ultimately aiming for consensus and better diagnostic accuracy. For more information, visit the Genome Connect website.

7. Conclusion

Looking forward, the establishment of regulatory standards, coupled with advancements in bioinformatic automation and AI-driven variant interpretation, will transform precision medicine [349]. Improved models that integrate genetic, biochemical, and clinical data will fill existing gaps in the early diagnosis and treatment of lysosomal diseases [350]. As these innovations continue to mature, they will lead to more effective personalized therapies, earlier interventions, and better overall patient outcomes.

Conflict of interest

None declared.

Author details

Irina Vlasova-St. Louis[1]*, Uri Barak[2] and Svetlana Khaiboullina[3]

1 Vinnana AI LLC, USA

2 Schneider Children's Medical Center of Israel, Israel

3 Kazan Federal University, Russia

*Address all correspondence to: stlouil@alumni.jh.edu

References

[1] Emms A, Castleman J, Allen S, Williams D, Kinning E, Kilby M. Next generation sequencing after invasive prenatal testing in fetuses with congenital malformations: Prenatal or neonatal investigation. Genes. 2022;**13**:1-9. DOI: 10.3390/genes13091517

[2] Ceyhan-Birsoy O, Murry JB, Machini K, Lebo MS, Yu TW, Fayer S, et al. Interpretation of genomic sequencing results in healthy and ill newborns: Results from the BabySeq project. American Journal of Human Genetics. 2019;**104**:76-93. DOI: 10.1016/j.ajhg.2018.11.016

[3] Kingsmore SF. Dispatches from Biotech beginning BeginNGS: Rapid newborn genome sequencing to end the diagnostic and therapeutic odyssey. American journal of medical genetics. Part C, Seminars in medical genetics. 2022;**190**:243-256. DOI: 10.1002/ajmg.c.32005

[4] Mansoor S, Qamar R, Azam M. Inborn errors of metabolism: Historical perspectives to contemporary management. Clinica Chimica Acta. 2024;**562**:119883. DOI: 10.1016/j.cca.2024.119883

[5] Marian AJ. Clinical interpretation and management of genetic variants. Journal of the American College of Cardiology. Basic to Translational Science. 2020;**5**:1029-1042. DOI: 10.1016/j.jacbts.2020.05.013

[6] Shen G, Li W, Zhang Y, Chen L. Next-generation sequencing based newborn screening and comparative analysis with MS/MS. BMC Pediatrics. 2024;**24**:230. DOI: 10.1186/s12887-024-04718-x

[7] Fung KW, Xu J, Bodenreider O. The new international classification of diseases 11th edition: A comparative analysis with ICD-10 and ICD-10-CM. Journal of the American Medical Informatics Association : JAMIA. 2020;**27**:738-746. DOI: 10.1093/jamia/ocaa030

[8] Ferreira CR, Rahman S, Keller M, Zschocke J, Abdenur J, Ali H, et al. An international classification of inherited metabolic disorders (ICIMD). Journal of Inherited Metabolic Disease. 2021;**44**:164-177. DOI: 10.1002/jimd.12348

[9] Kingma SDK, Bodamer OA, Wijburg FA. Epidemiology and diagnosis of lysosomal storage disorders; challenges of screening. Best Practice & Research. Clinical Endocrinology & Metabolism. 2015;**29**:145-157. DOI: 10.1016/j.beem.2014.08.004 [Accessed: January 9, 2024]

[10] Pastores GM. Lysosomal storage disorders: Clinical and therapeutic aspects. Handbook of Clinical Neurology. 2023;**196**:557-567. DOI: 10.1016/B978-0-323-98817-9.00006-5 [Accessed: January 9, 2024]

[11] Strovel ET, Cusmano-Ozog K, Wood T, Yu C. Measurement of lysosomal enzyme activities: A technical standard of the American College of Medical Genetics and Genomics (ACMG). Genetics in Medicine. 2022;**24**:769-783. DOI: 10.1016/j.gim.2021.12.013

[12] Li J, Mao S, Chao Y, Hu C, Qian Y, Dai Y, et al. Application of tandem mass spectrometry in the screening and diagnosis of mucopolysaccharidoses. Orphanet Journal of Rare Diseases. 2024;**19**:179. DOI: 10.1186/s13023-024-03195-w

[13] Li W, Cologna SM. Mass spectrometry-based proteomics in neurodegenerative lysosomal storage disorders. Molecular Omics. 2022;**18**:256-278. DOI: 10.1039/d2mo00004k

[14] Chuang C, Lee C, Tu R, Lo Y, Sisca F, Chang Y, et al. Nationwide newborn screening program for mucopolysaccharidoses in Taiwan and an update of the "Gold Standard" criteria required to make a confirmatory diagnosis. Diagnostics (Basel). 2021;**11**:1583. DOI: 10.3390/diagnostics11091583

[15] Elmonem MA, Abdelazim AM. Novel biomarkers for lysosomal storage disorders: Metabolomic and proteomic approaches. Clinica Chimica Acta. 2020;**509**:195-209. DOI: 10.1016/j.cca.2020.06.028

[16] Kim MJ, Kim SY, Lee JS, Kang S, Park L, Choi W, et al. Rapid targeted sequencing using dried blood spot samples for patients with suspected actionable genetic diseases. Annals of Laboratory Medicine. 2023;**43**:280-289. DOI: 10.3343/alm.2023.43.3.280 [Accessed: January 2, 2024]

[17] Wasserstein MP, Caggana M, Bailey SM, Desnick RJ, Edelmann L, Estrella L, et al. The New York pilot newborn screening program for lysosomal storage diseases: Report of the first 65,000 infants. Genetics in Medicine. 2019;**21**:631-640. DOI: 10.1038/s41436-018-0129-y

[18] Zanetti A, D'Avanzo F, Bertoldi L, Zampieri G, Feltrin E, De Pascale F, et al. Setup and validation of a targeted next-generation sequencing approach for the diagnosis of lysosomal storage disorders. The Journal of Molecular Diagnostics : JMD. 2020;**22**:488-502. DOI: 10.1016/j.jmoldx.2020.01.010

[19] Carter MT, Srour M, Au PB, Buhas D, Dyack S, Eaton A, et al. Genetic and metabolic investigations for neurodevelopmental disorders: Position statement of the Canadian College of Medical Geneticists (CCMG). Journal of Medical Genetics. 2023;**60**:523-532. DOI: 10.1136/jmg-2022-108962

[20] Jo YH, Choi SH, Yoo HW, Kwak MJ, Park KH, Kong J, et al. Clinical use of whole exome sequencing in children with developmental delay/intellectual disability. Pediatrics and Neonatology. 2024;**5**:445-450. DOI: 10.1016/j.pedneo.2023.05.015

[21] Jerves Serrano T, Gold J, Cooper JA, Church HJ, Tylee KL, Wu HY, et al. Hepatomegaly and splenomegaly: An approach to the diagnosis of lysosomal storage diseases. Journal of Clinical Medicine. 2024;**13**:1465. DOI: 10.3390/jcm13051465

[22] La Cognata V, Guarnaccia M, Morello G, Ruggieri M, Polizzi A, Cavallaro S. Design and validation of a custom NGS panel targeting a set of lysosomal storage diseases candidate for NBS applications. International Journal of Molecular Sciences. 2021;**22**:10064. DOI: 10.3390/ijms221810064

[23] La Cognata V, Cavallaro S. Detection of structural variants by NGS: Revealing missing alleles in lysosomal storage diseases. Biomedicine. 2022;**10**:1836. DOI: 10.3390/biomedicines10081836 [Accessed: December 29, 2023]

[24] Chang S, Zhan X, Liu Y, Song H, Gong Z, Han L, et al. Newborn screening for 6 lysosomal storage disorders in China. JAMA Network Open.

2024;**7**:e2410754. DOI: 10.1001/jamanetworkopen.2024.10754

[25] Stenton SL, Campagna M, Philippakis A, O'Donnell-Luria A, Gelb MH. First-tier next-generation sequencing for newborn screening: An important role for biochemical second-tier testing. Genetics in Medicine Open. 2023;**1**:100821. DOI: 10.1016/j.gimo.2023.100821

[26] Uribe-Carretero E, Rey V, Fuentes JM, Tamargo-Gómez I. Lysosomal dysfunction: Connecting the dots in the landscape of human diseases. Biology (Basel, Switzerland). 2024;**13**:34. DOI: 10.3390/biology13010034

[27] Fernández-Marmiesse A, Morey M, Pineda M, Eiris J, Couce ML, Castro-Gago M, et al. Assessment of a targeted resequencing assay as a support tool in the diagnosis of lysosomal storage disorders. Orphanet Journal of Rare Diseases. 2014;**9**:59. DOI: 10.1186/1750-1172-9-59

[28] Richards S, Aziz N, Bale S, Bick D, Das S, Gastier-Foster J, et al. Standards and guidelines for the interpretation of sequence variants: A joint consensus recommendation of the American College of Medical Genetics and Genomics and the Association for Molecular Pathology. Genetics in Medicine. 2015;**17**:405-424. DOI: 10.1038/gim.2015.30

[29] Ghosh R, Oak N, Plon SE. Evaluation of in silico algorithms for use with ACMG/AMP clinical variant interpretation guidelines. Genome Biology. 2017;**18**:225. DOI: 10.1186/s13059-017-1353-5

[30] Bean LJH, Hegde MR. Clinical implications and considerations for evaluation of in silico algorithms for use with ACMG/AMP clinical variant interpretation guidelines. Genome Medicine. 2017;**9**:111. DOI: 10.1186/s13073-017-0508-z

[31] Fang X, Zhu C, Zhu X, Feng Y, Jiao Z, Duan H, et al. Molecular analysis and novel variation identification of Chinese pedigrees with mucopolysaccharidosis using targeted next-generation sequencing. Clinica Chimica Acta. 2022;**524**:194-200. DOI: 10.1016/j.cca.2021.11.019

[32] Kumari A. Chapter 14 - Lipid Storage Disorders/Sphingolipidoses. Netherlands: Elsevier Inc.; 2023. pp. 93-104

[33] Dubot P, Sabourdy F, Levade T. Human genetic defects of sphingolipid synthesis. Journal of Inherited Metabolic Disease. 2024;**8**(1):1-15. DOI: 10.1002/jimd.12745

[34] Yagci ZB, Esvap E, Ozkara HA, Ulgen KO, Olmez EO. Inflammatory response and its relation to sphingolipid metabolism proteins: Chaperones as potential indirect anti-inflammatory agents. Advances in Protein Chemistry and Structural Biology. 2019;**114**:153-219. DOI: 10.1016/bs.apcsb.2018.09.004

[35] Sandhoff R, Sandhoff K. Neuronal ganglioside and glycosphingolipid (GSL) metabolism and disease: Cascades of secondary metabolic errors can generate complex pathologies (in LSDs). Glycobiology of the Nervous System. Cham: Springer; 2023;**29**:333-390. DOI: 10.1007/978-3-031-12390-0_12

[36] Abed Rabbo M, Khodour Y, Kaguni LS, Stiban J. Sphingolipid lysosomal storage diseases: From bench to bedside. Lipids in Health and Disease. 2021;**20**:44. DOI: 10.1186/s12944-021-01466-0

[37] Polo G, Burlina AP, Kolamunnage TB, Zampieri M, Dionisi-Vici C, Strisciuglio P,

et al. Diagnosis of sphingolipidoses: A new simultaneous measurement of lysosphingolipids by LC-MS/MS. Clinical Chemistry and Laboratory Medicine. 2017;**55**:403-414. DOI: 10.1515/cclm-2016-0340

[38] Iacono D, Koga S, Peng H, Manavalan A, Daiker J, Castanedes-Casey M, et al. Galactosylceramidase deficiency and pathological abnormalities in cerebral white matter of Krabbe disease. Neurobiology of Disease. 2022;**174**:105862. DOI: 10.1016/j.nbd.2022.105862

[39] Gowrishankar S, Cologna SM, Givogri MI, Bongarzone ER. Deregulation of signalling in genetic conditions affecting the lysosomal metabolism of cholesterol and galactosyl-sphingolipids. Neurobiology of Disease. 2020;**146**:105142. DOI: 10.1016/j.nbd.2020.105142

[40] Peterson L, Siemon A, Olewiler L, McBride KL, Allain DC. A qualitative assessment of parental experiences with false-positive newborn screening for Krabbe disease. Journal of Genetic Counseling. 2022;**31**:252-260. DOI: 10.1002/jgc4.1480

[41] Basheeruddin K, Shao R, Balster F, Gardley P, Ashbaugh L. Newborn screening for Krabbe disease—Illinois experience: Role of Psychosine in diagnosis of the disease. International Journal of Neonatal Screening. 2021;**7**:24. DOI: 10.3390/ijns7020024

[42] Orsini JJ, Kay DM, Saavedra-Matiz CA, Wenger DA, Duffner PK, Erbe RW, et al. Newborn screening for Krabbe disease in New York state: The first eight years' experience. Genetics in Medicine. 2016;**18**:239-248. DOI: 10.1038/gim.2015.211 [Accessed: January 7, 2024]

[43] Aerts-Kaya F, van Til N, P. Gene and Cellular therapies for leukodystrophies. Pharmaceutics. 2023;**15**:2522. DOI: 10.3390/pharmaceutics15112522

[44] Therrell BL, Padilla CD, Borrajo GJC, Khneisser I, Schielen PCJI, Knight-Madden J, et al. Current status of newborn bloodspot screening worldwide 2024: A comprehensive review of recent activities (2020-2023). International Journal of Neonatal Screening. 2024;**10**:38. DOI: 10.3390/ijns10020038

[45] Zhang X, Niu G, Song P, Wang L, Han R, Chu M, et al. Compound heterozygous pathogenic variants in the GALC gene cause infant-onset Krabbe disease. Translational Pediatrics. 2021;**10**:2552-2562. DOI: 10.21037/tp-21-403

[46] Hwang N, Kim S, Kim Y, Ha C, Lee J, Choi B, et al. Clinical feature, GALC variant spectrum, and genotype–phenotype correlation in Korean Krabbe disease patients: Multicenter experience over 13 years. Clinical Genetics. 2024;**106**:150-160. DOI: 10.1111/cge.14523

[47] Aslanger AD, Şengenç E, Kölemen AB, Demiral E, Alkan A, İşcan A, et al. Clinical and molecular findings in 6 Turkish cases with Krabbe disease. The Turkish Journal of Pediatrics. 2022;**64**:69-78. DOI: 10.24953/turkjped.2020.3713

[48] Corre CS, Matern D, Pellegrino JE, Saavedra-Matiz C, Orsini JJ, Thompson-Stone R. Low psychosine in Krabbe disease with onset in late infancy: A case report. International Journal of Neonatal Screening. 2021;**7**:28. DOI: 10.3390/ijns7020028

[49] Xia Z, Wenwen Y, Xianfeng Y, Panpan H, Xiaoqun Z, Zhongwu S. Adult-onset Krabbe disease due to a homozygous GALC mutation without abnormal signals on an MRI in a

consanguineous family: A case report. Molecular Genetics & Genomic Medicine. 2020;**8**:e1407. DOI: 10.1002/mgg3.1407

[50] Mächtel R, Dobert J, Hehr U, Weiss A, Kettwig M, Laugwitz L, et al. Late-onset Krabbe disease presenting as spastic paraplegia – Implications of GCase and CTSB/D. Annals of Clinical and Translational Neurology. 2024;**11**:1715-1731. DOI: 10.1002/acn3.52078

[51] Paiva ARB, Fonseca Neto RE, Afonso CL, Freua F, Nóbrega PR, Kok F. Incidental magnetic resonance imaging findings leading to an unusual diagnosis: Adult onset Krabbe disease. European Journal of Neurology. 2022;**29**:1859-1862. DOI: 10.1111/ene.15298

[52] Liu Y, Ma X, Chen Z, He R, Zhang Y, Dong H, et al. Dual rare genetic diseases in five pediatric patients: Insights from next-generation diagnostic methods. Orphanet Journal of Rare Diseases. 2024;**19**:159. DOI: 10.1186/s13023-024-03148-3

[53] Goldberg JD, Pierson S, Johansen Taber K. Expanded carrier screening: What conditions should we screen for? Prenatal Diagnosis. 2023;**43**:496-505. DOI: 10.1002/pd.6306

[54] Bennett LL. In: Bennett LL, editor. Gaucher's Disease : From Diagnosis to Treatment. New York: Nova Medicine & Health; 2020

[55] Goker-Alpan O, Ivanova MM. Neuronopathic Gaucher disease: Rare in the west, common in the east. Journal of Inherited Metabolic Disease. 2024;**47**(5):917-934. DOI: 10.1002/jimd.12749

[56] Vernet Machado Bressan Wilke M, Iop GD, Faqueti L, Lemos da Silva LA, Kubaski F, Poswar FO, et al. A Brazilian rare-disease center's experience with glucosylsphingosine (lyso-Gb1) in patients with Gaucher disease: Exploring a novel correlation with IgG levels in plasma and a biomarker measurement in CSF. International Journal of Molecular Sciences. 2024;**25**:2870. DOI: 10.3390/ijms25052870

[57] Daykin EC, Ryan E, Sidransky E. Diagnosing neuronopathic Gaucher disease: New considerations and challenges in assigning Gaucher phenotypes. Molecular Genetics and Metabolism. 2021;**132**:49-58. DOI: 10.1016/j.ymgme.2021.01.002

[58] Miyamoto T, Iino M, Komorizono Y, Kiguchi T, Furukawa N, Otsuka M, et al. Screening for Gaucher disease using dried blood spot tests: A Japanese multicenter, cross-sectional survey. Internal Medicine. 2021;**60**:699-707. DOI: 10.2169/internalmedicine.5064-20

[59] Lei K, Zhao Y, Sun L, Liang H, Luo R, Sun X, et al. A pilot screening of high-risk Gaucher disease children using dried blood spot methods in Shandong province of China. Orphanet Journal of Rare Diseases. 2018;**13**:48. DOI: 10.1186/s13023-018-0782-x

[60] Tang C, Jia X, Tang F, Liu S, Jiang X, Zhao X, et al. Detection of glucosylsphingosine in dried blood spots for diagnosis of Gaucher disease by LC-MS/MS. Clinical Biochemistry. 2021;**87**:79-84. DOI 10.1016/j.clinbiochem.2020.10.011

[61] Arevalo-Vargas I, Gonzalo IS, Lahoz C, Mozas P, Giraldo P, Aerts J. Exploring lipid biomarkers in Gaucher disease: LC-MS/MS analysis of dried blood spot samples. Molecular Genetics and Metabolism. 2024;**141**:107751. DOI: 10.1016/j.ymgme.2023.107751

[62] Chiong MAD, Racoma MJC, Abacan MAR. Genetic and clinical characteristics of Filipino patients with Gaucher disease. Molecular Genetics and Metabolism Reports. 2018;**15**:110-115. DOI: 10.1016/j.ymgmr.2018.03.010

[63] Granek Z, Barczuk J, Siwecka N, Rozpędek-Kamińska W, Kucharska E, Majsterek I. GBA1 gene mutations in α-synucleinopathies-molecularmechanisms underlying pathology and their clinical significance. International Journal of Molecular Sciences. 2023;**24**:2044. DOI: 10.3390/ijms24032044

[64] Zampieri S, Cattarossi S, Bembi B, Dardis A. GBA analysis in next-generation era: Pitfalls, challenges, and possible solutions. The Journal of Molecular Diagnostics : JMD. 2017;**19**:733-741. DOI: 10.1016/j.jmoldx.2017.05.005

[65] Velayati A, Knight MA, Stubblefield BK, Sidransky E, Tayebi N. Identification of recombinant alleles using quantitative real-time PCR implications for Gaucher disease. The Journal of Molecular Diagnostics : JMD. 2011;**13**:401-405. DOI: 10.1016/j.jmoldx.2011.02.005

[66] Woo EG, Tayebi N, Sidransky E. Next-generation sequencing analysis of GBA1: The challenge of detecting complex recombinant alleles. Frontiers in Genetics. 2021;**12**:684067. DOI: 10.3389/fgene.2021.684067

[67] Amico G, Grossi S, Vijzelaar R, Lanza F, Mazzotti R, Corsolini F, et al. MLPA-based approach for initial and simultaneous detection of GBA deletions and recombinant alleles in patients affected by Gaucher disease. Molecular Genetics and Metabolism. 2016;**119**:329-337. DOI: 10.1016/j.ymgme.2016.10.008

[68] Basgalupp SP, Siebert M, Vairo FPE, Chami AM, Pinto LLDC, Carvalho GDS, et al. Use of a multiplex ligation-dependent probe amplification method for the detection of deletions/duplications in the GBA1 gene in Gaucher disease patients. Blood Cells, Molecules, & Diseases. 2018;**68**:17-20. DOI: 10.1016/j.bcmd.2016.10.013

[69] Leija-Salazar M, Sedlazeck FJ, Toffoli M, Mullin S, Mokretar K, Athanasopoulou M, et al. Evaluation of the detection of GBA missense mutations and other variants using the Oxford Nanopore MinION. Molecular Genetics & Genomic Medicine. 2019;7:e564–n/a. DOI: 10.1002/mgg3.564

[70] Jeong S-Y, Park S-J, Kim HJ. Clinical and genetic characteristics of Korean patients with Gaucher disease. Blood Cells, Molecules, and Diseases. 2011;**46**:11-14. DOI: 10.1016/j.bcmd.2010.07.010

[71] Rossi C, Ferrante R, Valentinuzzi S, Zucchelli M, Buccolini C, Di Rado S, et al. Noninvasive DBS-based approaches to assist clinical diagnosis and treatment monitoring of Gaucher disease. Biomedicine. 2023;**11**:2672. DOI: 10.3390/biomedicines11102672

[72] Lepe-Balsalobre E, Santotoribio JD, Nuñez-Vazquez R, García-Morillo S, Jiménez-Arriscado P, Hernández-Arévalo P, et al. Genotype/phenotype relationship in Gaucher disease patients. Novel mutation in glucocerebrosidase gene. Clinical Chemistry and Laboratory Medicine (CCLM). 2020;**58**:2017-2024. DOI: 10.1515/cclm-2020-0306

[73] Gleason AM, D'Souza A, Ryan E, Grochowsky AR, Carter CR, Goker-Alpan O, et al. The D409H variant in GBA1: Challenges in predicting the Gaucher phenotype in the newborn screening era. American Journal of Medical Genetics. Part A. 2023;**191**:1783-1791. DOI: 10.1002/ajmg.a.63202

[74] Ryan E, Tayebi N, D'Souza A, Lopez G, Lichtenberg J, Sidransky E. Revisiting the diagnosis of Gaucher disease in a family with multiple GBA1 variants. American Journal of Medical Genetics. Part A. 2023;**191**:2647-2650. DOI: 10.1002/ajmg.a.63345

[75] Yang AC, Bier L, Overbey JR, Cohen-Pfeffer J, Desai K, Desnick RJ, et al. Early manifestations of type 1 Gaucher disease in presymptomatic children diagnosed after parental carrier screening. Genetics in Medicine. 2017;**19**:652-658. DOI: 10.1038/gim.2016.159

[76] Dardis A, Michelakakis H, Rozenfeld P, Fumic K, Wagner J, Pavan E, et al. Patient centered guidelines for the laboratory diagnosis of Gaucher disease type 1. Orphanet Journal of Rare Diseases. 2022;**17**:442. DOI: 10.1186/s13023-022-02573-6

[77] Weinreb NJ. The international cooperative Gaucher group (ICCG) Gaucher registry. Best Practice & Research. Clinical Haematology. 2023;**36**:101522. DOI: 10.1016/j.beha.2023.101522 [Accessed: January 9, 2024]

[78] Lu W, Chien Y, Tsai F, Hwu W, Chou Y, Chu S, et al. Changing clinical manifestations of Gaucher disease in Taiwan. Orphanet Journal of Rare Diseases. 2023;**18**:1-293. DOI: 10.1186/s13023-023-02895-z

[79] Vieira SRL, Schapira AHV. Glucocerebrosidase mutations and Parkinson disease. Journal of Neural Transmission. 2022;**129**:1105-1117. DOI: 10.1007/s00702-022-02531-3

[80] Gou P, Leng J, Cheng X, Zhang J. Clinical evaluation, accurate diagnosis and treatment of four pedigrees with Fabry's disease. Frontiers in Pediatrics. 2023;**11**:1057014. DOI: 10.3389/fped.2023.1057014

[81] Ortiz A, Germain DP, Desnick RJ, Politei J, Mauer M, Burlina A, et al. Fabry disease revisited: Management and treatment recommendations for adult patients. Molecular Genetics and Metabolism. 2018;**123**:416-427. DOI: 10.1016/j.ymgme.2018.02.014

[82] Tanaka K, Sugiyama H, Morinaga H, Onishi A, Tanabe K, Uchida HA, et al. Late-onset renal variant Fabry disease with R112H mutation and mild increase in plasma globotriaosylsphingosine: A case report. Frontiers in Medicine. 2024;**11**:1383309. DOI: 10.3389/fmed.2024.1383309

[83] Bossio S, Perrotta ID, Lofaro D, La Russa D, Rago V, Bonofiglio R, et al. The missense variant in the signal peptide of α-GLA gene, c.13 A/G, promotes endoplasmic reticular stress and the related pathway's activation. Genes. 2024;**15**:947. DOI: 10.3390/genes15070947

[84] Rodríguez Doyágüez P, Furlano M, Ars Criach E, Arce Y, Guirado L, Torra Balcells R. Correlation of X chromosome inactivation with clinical presentation of Fabry disease in a case report. Nefrología. 2023;**43**:91-95. DOI: 10.1016/j.nefroe.2024.01.018

[85] Harale M, Oommen AB, Mundada M, Faruqi AA, Patil S. An atypical presentation of Fabry disease in a patient with nephrotic syndrome: A case report. Curēus (Palo Alto, CA). 2024;**16**:e63661. DOI: 10.7759/cureus.63661

[86] Hitoshi Sakuraba H, Togawa T, Tsukimura T, Saito S. Comparative study on α-galactosidase A (GLA) genetic variants with unknown clinical significance. Molecular Genetics and

Metabolism. 2016;**117**:S100-S101. DOI: 10.1016/j.ymgme.2015.12.423

[87] Akeho N, Muta K, Torigoe K, Kitamura M, Sawada T, Nakamura K, et al. Cases of Fabry disease in which pathogenic variants are not detected in parent-child pairs. Curēus (Palo Alto, CA). 2024;**16**:e64127. DOI: 10.7759/cureus.64127

[88] Indennidate C, Faganello G, Sinagra G, Di Lenarda A. 641 A controversial case of Fabry disease: Adding another piece to the interpretation puzzle of c.376a>g missense mutation, a pathogenic variant. European Heart Journal Supplements. 2022;**24**. DOI: 10.1093/eurheartjsupp/suac121.625

[89] Riccio E, Pisani A. New insights in efficacy of different enzyme replacement therapy dosages in Fabry disease: Switch studies data following agalsidase beta shortage. Clinical Genetics. 2023;**103**:371-376. DOI: 10.1111/cge.14266

[90] Bichet DG, Hopkin RJ, Aguiar P, Allam SR, Chien Y, Giugliani R, et al. Consensus recommendations for the treatment and management of patients with Fabry disease on migalastat: A modified Delphi study. Frontiers in Medicine. 2023;**10**:1220637. DOI: 10.3389/fmed.2023.1220637

[91] Yu FPS, Amintas S, Levade T, Medin JA. Acid ceramidase deficiency: Farber disease and SMA-PME. Orphanet Journal of Rare Diseases. 2018;**13**:121-119. DOI: 10.1186/s13023-018-0845-z

[92] Puma A, Ezaru A, Cavalli M, Villa L, Torre F, Biancalana V, et al. A case of ASAH1-related pure SMA evolving into adult-onset Farber disease. Clinical Genetics. 2021;**100**:234-235. DOI: 10.1111/cge.13974

[93] Lee BH, Mongiovi P, Levade T, Marston B, Mountain J, Ciafaloni E. Spinal muscular atrophy and Farber disease due to ASAH1 variants: A case report. American Journal of Medical Genetics. Part A. 2020;**182**:2369-2371. DOI: 10.1002/ajmg.a.61764

[94] Mahmoud IG, Elmonem MA, Zaki MS, Ramadan A, Al-Menabawy NM, El-Gamal A, et al. ASAH1-related disorders: Description of 15 novel pediatric patients and expansion of the clinical phenotype. Clinical Genetics. 2020;**98**:598-605. DOI: 10.1111/cge.13834

[95] Najafi A, Tasharrofi B, Zandsalimi F, Rasulinezhad M, Ghahvechi Akbari M, Zamani G, et al. Spinal muscular atrophy with progressive myoclonic epilepsy (SMA-PME): Three new cases and review of the mutational spectrum. Italian Journal of Pediatrics. 2023;**49**:64. DOI: 10.1186/s13052-023-01474-z

[96] Wander A, Meena AK, Ghangoriya PK, Chakrabarty B, Jauhari P, Gulati S. ASAH1 variants causing spinal muscular atrophy phenotype. Indian Journal of Pediatrics. 2023;**91**(12):1274-1277. DOI: 10.1007/s12098-023-04957-3

[97] Karimzadeh P, Najmabadi H, Lochmuller H, Babaee M, Dehdahsi S, Miryounesi M, et al. Five patients with spinal muscular atrophy-progressive myoclonic epilepsy (SMA-PME): A novel pathogenic variant, treatment and review of the literature. Neuromuscular Disorders : NMD. 2022;**32**:806-810. DOI: 10.1016/j.nmd.2022.08.002

[98] Lee MM, McDowell GSV, De Vivo DC, Friedman D, Berkovic SF, Spanou M, et al. The clinical spectrum of SMA-PME and in vitro normalization of its cellular ceramide profile. Annals of Clinical and Translational Neurology.

2022;**9**:1941-1952. DOI: 10.1002/acn3.51687

[99] Zielonka M, Garbade SF, Kölker S, Hoffmann GF, Ries M. A cross-sectional quantitative analysis of the natural history of Farber disease: An ultra-orphan condition with rheumatologic and neurological cardinal disease features. Genetics in Medicine. 2018;**20**:524-530. DOI: 10.1038/gim.2017.133

[100] Alves MQ, Le Trionnaire E, Ribeiro I, Carpentier S, Harzer K, Levade T, et al. Molecular basis of acid ceramidase deficiency in a neonatal form of Farber disease: Identification of the first large deletion in ASAH1 gene. Molecular Genetics and Metabolism. 2013;**109**:276-281. DOI: 10.1016/j.ymgme.2013.04.019

[101] Thomas JA, Lam C, Berry GT. 23 - Lysosomal Storage, Peroxisomal, and Glycosylation Disorders and Smith–Lemli–Opitz Syndrome Presenting in the Neonate. Netherlands: Elsevier Inc; 2018. pp. 253-272.e3

[102] Oktay EO. Bioinformatics analysis of functional SNPs in human ASAH1 gene related to Farber disease. Russian Journal of Genetics. 2022;**58**:109-115. DOI: 10.1134/S1022795422010070

[103] Yan S, Fu F, Zhou H, Huang R, Wang Y, Liao C. Functional analysis of a novel splice site variant in the ASAH1 gene. Molecular Genetics & Genomic Medicine. 2024;**12**:e2317. DOI: 10.1002/mgg3.2317

[104] Kleynerman A, Rybova J, Faber ML, McKillop WM, Levade T, Medin JA. Acid ceramidase deficiency: Bridging gaps between clinical presentation, mouse models, and future therapeutic interventions. Biomolecules (Basel, Switzerland). 2023;**13**:274. DOI: 10.3390/biom13020274

[105] Eichler F, Sevin C, Barth M, Pang F, Howie K, Walz M, et al. Understanding caregiver descriptions of initial signs and symptoms to improve diagnosis of metachromatic leukodystrophy. Orphanet Journal of Rare Diseases. 2022;**17**:1-370. DOI: 10.1186/s13023-022-02518-z

[106] Issa AB, Feki FK, Jdila MB, Khabou B, Rhouma BB, Ammar-Keskes L, et al. Clinical, molecular, and computational analysis showed a novel homozygous mutation among the substrate-binding site of ARSA protein in consanguineous family with late-infantile MLD. Journal of Molecular Neuroscience. 2018;**66**:17-25. DOI: 10.1007/s12031-018-1141-z

[107] Gajbhiye V, Lamture Y, Uke P. Infantile metachromatic leukodystrophy (MLD): A rare case. Curēus (Palo Alto, CA). 2022;**14**:e33155. DOI: 10.7759/cureus.33155

[108] Doherty K, Frazier SB, Clark M, Childers A, Pruthi S, Wenger DA, et al. A closer look at ARSA activity in a patient with metachromatic leukodystrophy. Molecular Genetics and Metabolism Reports. 2019;**19**:100460. DOI: 10.1016/j.ymgmr.2019.100460

[109] Mir YR, Agrahari AK, Hassan A, Choudhary A, Asthana S, Taneja AK, et al. Identification and structural characterization of a pathogenic ARSA missense variant in two consanguineous families from Jammu and Kashmir (India) with late infantile metachromatic leukodystrophy. Molecular Biology Reports. 2024;**51**:30. DOI: 10.1007/s11033-023-09072-2

[110] Xu L, Zhong M, Wang Y, Wang Z, Song J, Zhao J, et al. Case report: Novel arylsulfatase A (ARSA) gene mutations in a patient with adult-onset metachromatic Leukodystrophy misdiagnosed as multiple sclerosis.

Frontiers in Neurology. 2021;**11**:576881. DOI: 10.3389/fneur.2020.576881

[111] Wang B, Lu F, Sun Y, Wang H. Case report: A compound heterozygous mutations in ARSA associated with adult-onset metachromatic leukodystrophy. Frontiers in Neurology. 2022;**13**:1011019. DOI: 10.3389/fneur.2022.1011019

[112] Wang Y, Chen X, Liu C, Wu S, Xie Q, Hu Q, et al. Metachromatic leukodystrophy: Characterization of two (p.Leu433Val, p.Gly449Arg) arylsulfatase A mutations. Experimental and Therapeutic Medicine. 2019;**18**:1738-1744. DOI: 10.3892/etm.2019.7760

[113] Beerepoot S, van Dooren SJM, Salomons GS, Boelens JJ, Jacobs EH, van der Knaap MS, et al. Metachromatic leukodystrophy genotypes in the Netherlands reveal novel pathogenic ARSA variants in non-Caucasian patients. Neurogenetics. 2020;**21**:289-299. DOI: 10.1007/s10048-020-00621-6

[114] Ben Issa A, Kamoun F, Bouchaala W, Charfi Triki C, Fakhfakh F. Complex genotypes in family with metachromatic leukodystrophy: Effect of trans and cis mutations distribution on the phenotype variability. International Journal of Developmental Neuroscience. 2024;**84**:35-46. DOI: 10.1002/jdn.10306

[115] Ataei Z, Nouri Z, Tavakoli F, Pourreza MR, Narrei S, Tabatabaiefar MA. Novel in-frame duplication variant characterization in late infantile metachromatic leukodystrophy using whole-exome sequencing and molecular dynamics simulation. PLoS One. 2023;**18**:e0282304. DOI: 10.1371/journal.pone.0282304

[116] Pekgül F, Eroğlu-Ertuğrul NG, Bekircan-Kurt C, Erdem-Ozdamar S, Çetinkaya A, Tan E, et al. Comprehensive clinical, biochemical, radiological and genetic analysis of 28 Turkish cases with suspected metachromatic leukodystrophy and their relatives. Molecular Genetics and Metabolism Reports. 2020;**25**:100688. DOI: 10.1016/j.ymgmr.2020.100688

[117] Cesani M, Lorioli L, Grossi S, Amico G, Fumagalli F, Spiga I, et al. Mutation update of ARSA and PSAP genes causing metachromatic leukodystrophy. Human Mutation. 2016;**37**:16-27. DOI: 10.1002/humu.22919

[118] Trinidad M, Hong X, Froelich S, Daiker J, Sacco J, Nguyen HP, et al. Predicting disease severity in metachromatic leukodystrophy using protein activity and a patient phenotype matrix. Genome Biology. 2023;**24**:172. DOI: 10.1186/s13059-023-03001-z

[119] Adang LA, Bonkowsky JL, Boelens JJ, Mallack E, Ahrens-Nicklas R, Bernat JA, et al. Consensus guidelines for the monitoring and management of metachromatic leukodystrophy in the United States. Cytotherapy (Oxford, England). 2024;**26**:739-748. DOI: 10.1016/j.jcyt.2024.03.487

[120] Wu THY, Brown HA, Church HJ, Kershaw CJ, Hutton R, Egerton C, et al. Improving newborn screening test performance for metachromatic leukodystrophy: Recommendation from a pre-pilot study that identified a late-infantile case for treatment. Molecular Genetics and Metabolism. 2024;**142**:108349. DOI: 10.1016/j.ymgme.2024.108349

[121] Schoenmakers DH, Mochel F, Adang LA, Boelens J, Calbi V, Eklund EA, et al. Inventory of current practices regarding hematopoietic stem cell transplantation in metachromatic leukodystrophy in Europe and neighboring countries. Orphanet

Journal of Rare Diseases. 2024;**19**:46. DOI: 10.1186/s13023-024-03075-3

[122] Beerepoot S, Boelens JJ, Lindemans C, de Witte MA, Nierkens S, Vrancken AFJE, et al. Progressive demyelinating polyneuropathy after hematopoietic cell transplantation in metachromatic leukodystrophy: A case series. Journal of Neurology. 2024;**271**:4028-4038. DOI: 10.1007/s00415-024-12322-3

[123] Zhang Z, Jiang H, Huang L, Liu S, Zhou X, Cai Y, et al. Lentivirus-modified hematopoietic stem cell gene therapy for advanced symptomatic juvenile metachromatic leukodystrophy: A long-term follow-up pilot study. Protein & Cell. 2024;**16**(1):16-27. DOI: 10.1093/procel/pwae037

[124] Sun Y, Witte DP, Zamzow M, Ran H, Quinn B, Matsuda J, et al. Combined saposin C and D deficiencies in mice lead to a neuronopathic phenotype, glucosylceramide and α-hydroxy ceramide accumulation, and altered prosaposin trafficking. Human Molecular Genetics. 2007;**16**:957-971. DOI: 10.1093/hmg/ddm040

[125] Bhat V, Thergaonkar RW, Thakur M, Rajkamal T. Combined saposin deficiency: A rare occurrence. Medical Journal. Armed Forces India. 2023;**79**:238-240. DOI: 10.1016/j.mjafi.2021.01.024

[126] Liaqat K, Hussain S, Acharya A, Nasir A, Bharadwaj T, Ansar M, et al. Phenotype expansion for atypical Gaucher disease due to homozygous missense PSAP variant in a large consanguineous Pakistani family. Genes. 2022;**13**:662. DOI: 10.3390/genes13040662

[127] Nair S, Bar N, Xu ML, Dhodapkar M, Mistry PK. Glucosyl-sphingosine but not Saposin C, is the target antigen in Gaucher disease-associated gammopathy. Molecular Genetics and Metabolism. 2020;**129**:286-291. DOI: 10.1016/j.ymgme.2020.01.009

[128] Zhu L, Zhang X, Guan Y, Zhu Y, Zhou Q, Liu B, et al. Meta-analysis of the association of prosaposin polymorphisms rs4747203 and rs885828 with risk of Parkinson's disease. Acta Neurologica Belgica. 2024;**124**:573-580. DOI: 10.1007/s13760-023-02446-0

[129] Kuo M, Chu Y, Su Y, Chen M, Wu R. Prosaposin variants in sporadic, familial, and early-onset Parkinson's disease: A Taiwanese case-control study and meta-analysis. Scientific Reports. 2024;**14**:2225. DOI: 10.1038/s41598-024-51646-y

[130] Breiden B, Sandhoff K. Lysosomal glycosphingolipid storage diseases. Annual Review of Biochemistry. 2019;**88**:461-485. DOI: 10.1146/annurev-biochem-013118-111518

[131] Karimzadeh P, Ebrahimi M, Etemad K, Ahmad Abadi F, Hosseini Nezhad Z. GM1 and GM2-gangliosidosis: Clinical features, neuroimaging findings and electroencephalography. Iranian Journal of Child Neurology. 2024;**18**:127-140. DOI: 10.22037/ijcn.v18i2.40751

[132] Godbole NP, Haxton E, Rowe OE, Locascio JJ, Schmahmann JD, Eichler FS, et al. Clinical and imaging predictors of late-onset GM2 gangliosidosis: A scoping review. Annals of Clinical and Translational Neurology. 2024;**11**:207-224. DOI: 10.1002/acn3.51947

[133] Foster D, Williams L, Arnold N, Larsen J. Therapeutic developments for neurodegenerative GM1 gangliosidosis. Frontiers in Neuroscience. 2024;**18**:1392683. DOI: 10.3389/fnins.2024.1392683

[134] Qureshi N, Hussein N, Henneman L, Kai J, Qureshi N. Preconception risk assessment for thalassaemia, sickle cell disease, cystic fibrosis and Tay-Sachs disease. Cochrane Database of Systematic Reviews. 2021;**2021**:CD010849. DOI: 10.1002/14651858.CD010849.pub4

[135] Nicoli E, Annunziata I, d'Azzo A, Platt FM, Tifft CJ, Stepien KM. GM1 gangliosidosis—A mini-review. Frontiers in Genetics. 2021;**12**:734878. DOI: 10.3389/fgene.2021.734878

[136] Noh ES, Park HM, Kim MS, Park H, Cho SY, Jin D. Late-infantile GM1 gangliosidosis: A case report. Medicine (Baltimore). 2022;**101**:e28435. DOI: 10.1097/MD.0000000000028435

[137] Rha AK, Maguire AS, Martin DR. GM1 Gangliosidosis: Mechanisms and management. Application of Clinical Genetics. 2021;**14**:209-233. DOI: 10.2147/TACG.S206076

[138] Guo Z. Ganglioside GM1 and the central nervous system. International Journal of Molecular Sciences. 2023;**24**:9558. DOI: 10.3390/ijms24119558

[139] Kern J, Böhringer J, Timmann D, Trollmann R, Stendel C, Kamm C, et al. Clinical, imaging, genetic, and disease course characteristics in patients with GM2 Gangliosidosis: Beyond age of onset. Neurology. 2024;**102**:e207898. DOI: 10.1212/WNL.0000000000207898

[140] Park JH, Ko JM, Kim MS, Kim MJ, Seong M, Yoo T, et al. Novel HEXA variants in Korean children with Tay–Sachs disease with regression of neurodevelopment from infancy. Molecular Genetics & Genomic Medicine. 2021;**9**:e1677. DOI: 10.1002/mgg3.1677

[141] Kissell J, Rochmann C, Minini P, Eichler F, Stephen CD, Lau H, et al. Clinical outcome assessments of disease burden and progression in late-onset GM2 gangliosidoses. Molecular Genetics and Metabolism. 2024;**142**:108512. DOI: 10.1016/j.ymgme.2024.108512

[142] Cheema HA, Waheed N, Saeed A. Unusual case of juvenile Tay-Sachs disease. BMJ Case Reports. 2019;**12**:e230140. DOI: 10.1136/bcr-2019-230140

[143] Sutton VR. Tay-Sachs disease: Screening and counseling families at risk for metabolic disease. Obstetrics and Gynecology Clinics of North America. 2002;**29**:287-296. DOI: 10.1016/S0889-8545(01)00002-X

[144] Ibrahim DMA, Ali OSM, Nasr H, Fateen E, AbdelAleem A. Biochemical and mutational analyses of HEXA in a cohort of Egyptian patients with infantile Tay-Sachs disease. Expansion of the mutation spectrum. Orphanet Journal of Rare Diseases. 2023;**18**:52. DOI: 10.1186/s13023-023-02637-1

[145] Mistri M, Mehta S, Solanki D, Kamate M, Gupta N, Kabra M, et al. Identification of novel variants in a large cohort of children with Tay–Sachs disease: An initiative of a multicentric task force on lysosomal storage disorders by Government of India. Journal of Human Genetics. 2019;**64**:985-994. DOI: 10.1038/s10038-019-0647-8

[146] Gu X, Kovacs AS, Myung Y, Ascher DB. Mutations in glycosyltransferases and Glycosidases: Implications for associated diseases. Biomolecules (Basel, Switzerland). 2024;**14**:497. DOI: 10.3390/biom14040497

[147] Gregg AR, Aarabi M, Klugman S, Leach NT, Bashford MT, Goldwaser T, et al. Screening for autosomal recessive

and X-linked conditions during pregnancy and preconception: A practice resource of the American College of Medical Genetics and Genomics (ACMG). Genetics in Medicine. 2021;**23**:1793-1806. DOI: 10.1038/s41436-021-01203-z

[148] Tropak MB, Yonekawa S, Karumuthil-Melethil S, Thompson P, Wakarchuk W, Gray SJ, et al. Construction of a hybrid β-hexosaminidase subunit capable of forming stable homodimers that hydrolyze GM2 ganglioside in vivo. Molecular Therapy. Methods & Clinical Development. 2016;**3**:15057. DOI: 10.1038/mtm.2015.57

[149] Toro C, Zainab M, Tifft CJ. The GM2 gangliosidoses: Unlocking the mysteries of pathogenesis and treatment. Neuroscience Letters. 2021;**764**:136195. DOI: 10.1016/j.neulet.2021.136195

[150] Yin J, Hu W, Huang Y. Clinical and genetic features of a case with juvenile onset sandhoff disease. BMC Neurology. 2023;**23**:240. DOI: 10.1186/s12883-023-03267-7

[151] Xie H, Lin S, Chen Y, Wang W, Qi Y, Li J, et al. A case of Sandhoff disease caused by a novel β-hexosaminidase B (HEXB) mutation c.118delG (p.A40fs24): A case report from China. Medicine (Baltimore). 2023;**102**:e33890. DOI: 10.1097/MD.0000000000033890

[152] Singer HS, Mink JW, Gilbert DL, Jankovic J. Chapter 17 - Metabolic Disorders with Associated Movement Abnormalities. Netherlands: Elsevier Inc; 2022. pp. 443-533

[153] Sung AR, Moretti P, Shaibani A. Case of late-onset Sandhoff disease due to a novel mutation in the HEXB gene. Neurology. Genetics. 2018;**4**:e260. DOI: 10.1212/NXG.0000000000000260

[154] Beecher G, Liewluck T, Milone M. Adult-onset Sandhoff disease in a Filipino patient: Asymmetric weakness, whole HEXB gene deletion, and coexisting MYH7 pathogenic variant. Neurology. Genetics. 2022;**8**:e672. DOI: 10.1212/NXG.0000000000000672

[155] Gowda VK, Gupta P, Bharathi NK, Bhat M, Shivappa SK, Benakappa N. Clinical and laboratory profile of Gangliosidosis from southern part of India. Journal of Pediatric Genetics (Birmingham, Ala.). 2022;**11**:34. DOI: 10.1055/s-0040-1718726

[156] Aureli M, Mauri L, Carsana EV, Dobi D, Breviario S, Lunghi G, et al. Gangliosides and Cell Surface Ganglioside Metabolic Enzymes in the Nervous System. Vol. 29. Switzerland: Springer International Publishing AG; 2023. pp. 305-332

[157] Cachon-Gonzalez M, Zaccariotto E, Cox TM. Genetics and therapies for GM2 Gangliosidosis. Current Gene Therapy. 2018;**18**:68-89. DOI: 10.2174/1566523218666180404162622

[158] Ganne B, Dauriat B, Richard L, Lamari F, Ghorab K, Magy L, et al. GM2 gangliosidosis AB variant: First case of late onset and review of the literature. Neurological Sciences. 2022;**43**:6517-6527. DOI: 10.1007/s10072-022-06270-x

[159] Ries M, Mendoza G, Arash-Kaps L, Amraoui Y, Quack F, Hardt B, et al. Quantitative longitudinal natural history of 8 gangliosidoses—Conceptual framework and baseline data of the German 8-in-1 disease registry. A cross-sectional analysis. Genetics in Medicine. 2022;**24**:2434-2443. DOI: 10.1016/j.gim.2022.09.001

[160] İnci A, Cengiz Ergin FB, Biberoğlu G, Okur İ, Ezgü FS, Tümer L. Two patients from Turkey with a novel

variant in the GM2A gene and review of the literature. Journal of Pediatric Endocrinology & Metabolism. 2021;**34**:805-812. DOI: 10.1515/jpem-2020-0655

[161] Brackmann F, Kehrer C, Kustermann W, Böhringer J, Krägeloh-Mann I, Trollmann R. Rare variant of GM2 gangliosidosis through activator-protein deficiency. Neuropediatrics. 2017;**48**:127-130. DOI: 10.1055/s-0037-1598646

[162] Bibi F, Ullah A, Bourinaris T, Efthymiou S, Kriouile Y, Sultan T, et al. Tay-Sachs disease: Two novel rare HEXA mutations from Pakistan and Morocco. Klinische Pädiatrie. 2021;**233**:226-230. DOI: 10.1055/a-1371-1561

[163] Gordon-Lipkin E, Cohen JS, Srivastava S, Soares BP, Levey E, Fatemi A. ST3GAL5-related disorders: A deficiency in ganglioside metabolism and a genetic cause of intellectual disability and choreoathetosis. Journal of Child Neurology. 2018;**33**:825-831. DOI: 10.1177/0883073818791099

[164] Quinville BM, Deschenes NM, Ryckman AE, Walia JS. A comprehensive review: Sphingolipid metabolism and implications of disruption in sphingolipid homeostasis. International Journal of Molecular Sciences. 2021;**22**:5793. DOI: 10.3390/ijms22115793

[165] Rudy N, Aoki K, Ananth A, Holloway L, Skinner C, Hurst A, et al. Compound heterozygous variants within two conserved sialyltransferase motifs of ST3GAL5 cause GM3 synthase deficiency. JIMD Reports. 2023;**64**:138-145. DOI: 10.1002/jmd2.12353

[166] Wang H, Wang A, Wang D, Bright A, Sency V, Zhou A, et al. Early growth and development impairments in patients with ganglioside GM3 synthase deficiency. Clinical Genetics. 2016;**89**:625-629. DOI: 10.1111/cge.12703

[167] Wang AS, Kilbane C. Dystonia Due to GM3 Synthase Deficiency. Movement Disorders Clinical Practice. Vol. 9. Hoboken, N.J, USA; 2022. pp. 236-239. DOI: 10.1002/mdc3.13399

[168] Heide S, Jacquemont M, Cheillan D, Renouil M, Tallot M, Schwartz CE, et al. GM3 synthase deficiency in non-Amish patients. Genetics in Medicine. 2022;**24**:492-498. DOI: 10.1016/j.gim.2021.10.007

[169] Indellicato R, Parini R, Domenighini R, Malagolini N, Iascone M, Gasperini S, et al. Total loss of GM3 synthase activity by a normally processed enzyme in a novel variant and in all ST3GAL5 variants reported to cause a distinct congenital disorder of glycosylation. Glycobiology (Oxford). 2019;**29**:229-241. DOI: 10.1093/glycob/cwy112

[170] Manoochehri J, Dastgheib SA, Khamirani HJ, Mollaie M, Sharifi Z, Zoghi S, et al. A novel frameshift pathogenic variant in ST3GAL5 causing salt and pepper developmental regression syndrome (SPDRS): A case report. Human Genome Variation. 2021;**8**:33. DOI: 10.1038/s41439-021-00164-8

[171] Abdulkareem AA, Shirah BH, Naseer MI. Whole exome sequencing reveals a novel homozygous variant in the ganglioside biosynthetic enzyme, ST3GAL5 gene in a Saudi family causing salt and pepper syndrome. Genes. 2023;**14**:1-9. DOI: 10.3390/genes14020354

[172] Watanabe S, Lei M, Nakagawa E, Takeshita E, Inamori K, Shishido F, et al. Neurological insights on two siblings with GM3 synthase deficiency due to novel compound heterozygous ST3GAL5

variants. Brain & Development (Tokyo 1979). 2023;**45**:270-277. DOI: 10.1016/j.braindev.2023.01.002

[173] Hosseini K, Fallahi J, Razban V, Sirat RZ, Varasteh M, Tarhriz V. Overview of clinical, molecular, and therapeutic features of Niemann–Pick disease (types A, B, and C): Focus on therapeutic approaches. Cell Biochemistry and Function. 2024;**42**:e4028. DOI: 10.1002/cbf.4028

[174] Pulikottil-Jacob R, Dehipawala S, Smith B, Athavale A, Gusto G, Chandak A, et al. Survival of patients with chronic acid sphingomyelinase a deficiency (ASMD) in the United States: A retrospective chart review study. Molecular Genetics and Metabolism Reports. 2024;**38**:101040. DOI: 10.1016/j.ymgmr.2023.101040

[175] Schuchman EH, Desnick RJ. Types A and B Niemann-Pick disease. Molecular Genetics and Metabolism. 2017;**120**:27-33. DOI: 10.1016/j.ymgme.2016.12.008

[176] Kang H, Zhou M, Xie C, Lu K. A 2-bp deletion mutation in SMPD1 gene leading to lysosomal acid sphingomyelinase deficiency in a Chinese consanguineous pedigree. Journal of Pediatric Endocrinology & Metabolism. 2022;**35**:1113-1116. DOI: 10.1515/jpem-2021-0480

[177] Wang R, Qin Z, Huang L, Luo H, Peng H, Zhou X, et al. SMPD1 expression profile and mutation landscape help decipher genotype–phenotype association and precision diagnosis for acid sphingomyelinase deficiency. Hereditas. 2023;**160**:11. DOI: 10.1186/s41065-023-00272-1

[178] Nasereddin A, Ereqat S. Deep sequencing of *SMPD1* gene revealed a heterozygous frameshift mutation (p.Ser192Alafs) in a Palestinian infant with Niemann–Pick disease type A: A case report. Journal of Medical Case Reports. 2018;**12**:272. DOI: 10.1186/s13256-018-1805-x

[179] Kavčič A, Homan M, Živanović M, Debeljak M, Butenko T, Drole Torkar A, et al. Compound heterozygote mutation in the SMPD1 gene leading to Nieman-Pick disease type A. The American Journal of Case Reports. 2022;**23**:e937220. DOI: 10.12659/AJCR.937220

[180] Zahedi Abghari F, Bayat F, Razipour M, Karimipoor M, Taghavi-Basmenj M, Zeinali S, et al. Characterization of Niemann-Pick diseases genes mutation spectrum in Iran and identification of a novel mutation in SMPD1 gene. Medical Journal of the Islamic Republic of Iran. 2019;**33**:126. DOI: 10.34171/mjiri.33.126

[181] Alipouran F, Ghayoor Karimiani E, Khayatzadeh J. Evaluation of the genetic background of patients with Niemann-Pick disease. Reports of Biochemistry And Molecular Biology. 2023;**12**:386-392. DOI: 10.61186/rbmb.12.3.386

[182] Ding Y, Li X, Liu Y, Hua Y, Song J, Wang L, et al. Seven novel mutations of the SMPD1 gene in four Chinese patients with Niemann-Pick disease type A and prenatal diagnosis for four fetuses. European Journal of Medical Genetics. 2016;**59**:263-268. DOI: 10.1016/j.ejmg.2015.11.012

[183] Al Shahrani AM, Asiri W, Alqarni SAM, Al Murayeh LM. Novel mutation in chromosome 11p15.4 causing Niemann-Pick disease type A in a Saudi child. Curēus (Palo Alto, CA). 2024;**16**:e55883. DOI: 10.7759/cureus.55883

[184] Gul F, Begum S, Rasool P, Shah S, Waqar M. A rare case of Niemann-Pick

disease Type-A. Curēus (Palo Alto, CA). 2024;**16**:e59427. DOI: 10.7759/cureus.59427

[185] Affendi LMN, Noor S, Binti A, Tong CV, Nordin NDB. Niemann-Pick disease with bilateral adrenal mass. JCEM Case Reports. 2023;**1**:luad152. DOI: 10.1210/jcemcr/luad152

[186] Cerón-Rodríguez M, Vázquez-Martínez ER, García-Delgado C, Ortega-Vázquez A, Valencia-Mayoral P, Ramírez-Devars L, et al. Niemann-Pick disease A or B in four pediatric patients and SMPD1 mutation carrier frequency in the Mexican population. Annals of Hepatology. 2019;**18**:613-619. DOI: 10.1016/j.aohep.2018.12.004

[187] Zhou Z, Wang S, Xu C, Wu W, Hui T, Yin Q, et al. Three-years misdiagnosis of Niemann Pick disease type B with novel mutations in SMPD1 gene as Budd-Chiari syndrome. BMC Medical Genomics. 2022;**15**:1-196. DOI: 10.1186/s12920-022-01353-2

[188] Wu F, Su D, Wang W, Song X, Fan S, Su J, et al. Case report: Clinical, imaging, and genetic characteristics of type B Niemann Pick disease combined with segawa syndrome diagnosed via dual gene sequencing. Frontiers in Genetics. 2024;**15**:1391936. DOI: 10.3389/fgene.2024.1391936

[189] Ordieres-Ortega L, Galeano-Valle F, Mallén-Pérez M, Muñoz-Delgado C, Apaza-Chavez J, Menárguez-Palanca FJ, et al. Niemann-Pick disease type-B: A unique case report with compound heterozygosity and complicated lipid management. BMC Medical Genetics. 2020;**21**:94. DOI: 10.1186/s12881-020-01027-9

[190] Giacomarra M, Colomba P, Francofonte D, Zora M, Caocci G, Diomede D, et al. Gaucher disease or acid sphingomyelinase deficiency? The importance of differential diagnosis. Journal of Clinical Medicine. 2024;**13**:1487. DOI: 10.3390/jcm13051487

[191] Cappellini MD, Motta I, Barbato A, Giuffrida G, Manna R, Carubbi F, et al. Similarities and differences between Gaucher disease and acid sphingomyelinase deficiency: An algorithm to support the diagnosis. European Journal of Internal Medicine. 2023;**108**:81-84. DOI: 10.1016/j.ejim.2022.11.028

[192] Arslan N, Coker M, Gokcay GF, Kiykim E, Onenli Mungan HN, Ezgu F. Expert opinion on patient journey, diagnosis and clinical monitoring in acid sphingomyelinase deficiency in Turkey: A pediatric metabolic disease specialist's perspective. Frontiers in Pediatrics. 2023;**11**:1113422. DOI: 10.3389/fped.2023.1113422

[193] Hon YY, Zaidi A, Giffin A, Wang Y, Lei N, Hossain MN, et al. Regulatory news: Olipudase alfa-rpcp (Xenpozyme™) for treatment of non-central nervous system manifestations of acid sphingomyelinase deficiency (ASMD) in adult and pediatric patients—FDA approval summary. Journal of Inherited Metabolic Disease. 2024;**47**:575-577. DOI: 10.1002/jimd.12754

[194] Wasserstein MP, Lachmann R, Hollak C, Barbato A, Gallagher RC, Giugliani R, et al. Continued improvement in disease manifestations of acid sphingomyelinase deficiency for adults with up to 2 years of olipudase alfa treatment: Open-label extension of the ASCEND trial. Orphanet Journal of Rare Diseases. 2023;**18**:1-378. DOI: 10.1186/s13023-023-02983-0

[195] Geberhiwot T, Wasserstein M, Wanninayake S, Bolton SC, Dardis A,

Lehman A, et al. Consensus clinical management guidelines for acid sphingomyelinase deficiency (Niemann–Pick disease types A, B and A/B). Orphanet Journal of Rare Diseases. 2023;**18**:85. DOI: 10.1186/s13023-023-02686-6

[196] Pfrieger FW. The Niemann-Pick type diseases – A synopsis of inborn errors in sphingolipid and cholesterol metabolism. Progress in Lipid Research. 2023;**90**:101225. DOI: 10.1016/j.plipres.2023.101225

[197] Yoon H, Jeong J, Kim G, Lee HH, Jang S. The point mutation of the cholesterol trafficking membrane protein NPC1 may affect its proper function in more than a single step: Molecular dynamics simulation study. Computational Biology and Chemistry. 2022;**99**:107725. DOI: 10.1016/j.compbiolchem.2022.107725

[198] Yoon H, Jeong H, Lee HH, Jang S. Molecular dynamics study with mutation shows that N-terminal domain structural re-orientation in Niemann-Pick type C1 is required for proper alignment of cholesterol transport. Journal of Neurochemistry. 2021;**156**:967-978. DOI: 10.1111/jnc.15150

[199] Mohamed AA, Gan W, Babici D, Hagan V, Wald R, Swerdloff M. Supranuclear palsy as an initial presentation of the adult-onset Niemann-Pick Type C. Neurology International. 2024;**16**:561-566. DOI: 10.3390/neurolint16030042

[200] Las Heras M, Szenfeld B, Ballout RA, Buratti E, Zanlungo S, Dardis A, et al. Understanding the phenotypic variability in Niemann-Pick disease type C (NPC): A need for precision medicine. NPJ Genomic Medicine. 2023;**8**:21. DOI: 10.1038/s41525-023-00365-w

[201] Sheth J, Joseph JJ, Shah K, Muranjan M, Mistri M, Sheth F. Pulmonary manifestations in Niemann-Pick type C disease with mutations in NPC2 gene: Case report and review of literature. BMC Medical Genetics. 2017;**18**:5. DOI: 10.1186/s12881-017-0367-x

[202] Sghaier N, Younes S, Machraoui R, Younes S, Habib Sfar M. Niemann-Pick disease type C, a rare cause of pancytopenia: A case report. International Journal of Hematology and Therapy. 2018;**4**:13-15. DOI: 10.15436/2381-1404.18.1634

[203] Singh V, Randad K, Yadav P, Sawant T, Ansari Q. Neonatal presentation of Niemann-Pick disease type C2 - A rare case report. Anuradhapura Medical Journal. 2023;**17**:54-57. DOI: 10.4038/amj.v17i3.7770

[204] Chamova T, Kirov A, Guerguelt-cheva V, Todorov T, Bojinova V, Zhelyazkova S, et al. Clinical spectrum and genetic variability in Bulgarian patients with Niemann-Pick disease Type C. European Neurology. 2016;**75**:113-123. DOI: 10.1159/000444480

[205] Erickson RP. Do GWAS and studies of heterozygotes for NPC1 and/or NPC2 explain why NPC disease cases are so rare? Journal of Applied Genetics. 2018;**59**:441-447. DOI: 10.1007/s13353-018-0465-2

[206] Kubaski F, Burlina A, Polo G, Pereira D, Herbst ZM, Silva C, et al. Experience of the NPC Brazil network with a comprehensive program for the screening and diagnosis of Niemann-Pick disease Type C. International Journal of Neonatal Screening. 2022;**8**:39. DOI: 10.3390/ijns8030039

[207] Tao C, Zhao M, Zhang X, Hao J, Huo Q, Sun J, et al. Novel compound

heterozygous mutations of the NPC1 gene associated with Niemann-Pick disease type C: A case report and review of the literature. BMC Infectious Diseases. 2024;**24**:145. DOI: 10.1186/s12879-024-09025-5

[208] Zhang G, Yu F, Zhang K, Li F, Lyu Y, Gao M, et al. Niemann-Pick disease type C caused by NPC1 mutation in a case. Chung-Hua I Hsueh I Chuan Hsueh Tsa Chih. 2019;**36**:480-483. DOI: 10.3760/cma.j.issn.1003-9406.2019.05.016

[209] Seker Yilmaz B, Baruteau J, Rahim AA, Gissen P. Clinical and molecular features of early infantile Niemann Pick type C disease. International Journal of Molecular Sciences. 2020;**21**:5059. DOI: 10.3390/ijms21145059

[210] Terada C, Mirarchi F, Marino R, Eiroa H, Berensztein E. Molecular and functional study of pediatric patients with Niemann-Pick C in Argentina. Medicina. 2022;**82**:308

[211] Greenberg CR, Barnes JG, Kogan S, Seargeant LE. A rare case of Niemann–Pick disease type C without neurological involvement in a 66-year-old patient. Molecular Genetics and Metabolism Reports. 2015;**3**:18-20. DOI: 10.1016/j.ymgmr.2015.02.004

[212] Pintavorn P, Munie S, Munagapati S. Lamellar bodies in podocytes associated with compound heterozygous mutations for Niemann Pick type C1 mimicking Fabry disease, a case report. Canadian Journal of Kidney Health and Disease. 2022;**9**:20543581221124635. DOI: 10.1177/20543581221124635

[213] Al-Shamrani A, Al-Shamrani K, Mahfoudh AB, Mohamed AS, Mohamed S. A Niemann-Pick disease type C2 with severe pulmonary involvement and limited therapeutic options: A case report. Children (Basel). 2022;**9**:1811. DOI: 10.3390/children9121811

[214] Alavi A, Nafissi S, Shamshiri H, Nejad MM, Elahi E. Identification of mutation in NPC2 by exome sequencing results in diagnosis of Niemann–Pick disease type C. Molecular Genetics and Metabolism. 2013;**110**:139-144. DOI: 10.1016/j.ymgme.2013.05.019

[215] Pineda M, Walterfang M, Patterson MC. Miglustat in Niemann-Pick disease type C patients: A review. Orphanet Journal of Rare Diseases. 2018;**13**:140. DOI: 10.1186/s13023-018-0844-0

[216] van Gool R, Tucker-Bartley A, Yang E, Todd N, Guenther F, Goodlett B, et al. Targeting neurological abnormalities in lysosomal storage diseases. Trends in Pharmacological Sciences (Regular ed.). 2022;**43**:495-509. DOI: 10.1016/j.tips.2021.11.005

[217] Mengel E, Patterson MC, Da Riol RM, Del Toro M, Deodato F, Gautschi M, et al. Efficacy and safety of arimoclomol in Niemann-Pick disease type C: Results from a double-blind, randomised, placebo-controlled, multinational phase 2/3 trial of a novel treatment. Journal of Inherited Metabolic Disease. 2021;**44**:1463-1480. DOI: 10.1002/jimd.12428

[218] Ago Y, Rintz E, Musini KS, Ma Z, Tomatsu S. Molecular mechanisms in pathophysiology of mucopolysaccharidosis and prospects for innovative therapy. International Journal of Molecular Sciences. 2024;**25**:1113. DOI: 10.3390/ijms25021113

[219] Galimberti C, Madeo A, Di Rocco M, Fiumara A. Mucopoly-saccharidoses: Early diagnostic signs in infants and children. Italian Journal of

Pediatrics. 2018;**44**:133. DOI: 10.1186/s13052-018-0550-5

[220] Zhou J, Lin J, Leung WT, Wang L. A basic understanding of mucopolysaccharidosis: Incidence, clinical features, diagnosis, and management. Intractable & Rare Diseases Research. 2020;**9**:1-9. DOI: 10.5582/irdr.2020.01011

[221] Puckett Y, Mallorga-Hernández A, Montaño AM. Epidemiology of mucopolysaccharidoses (MPS) in United States: Challenges and opportunities. Orphanet Journal of Rare Diseases. 2021;**16**:241. DOI: 10.1186/s13023-021-01880-8. Available from: https://www.ncbi.nlm.nih.gov/pmc/articles/PMC8164808/ [Accessed: January 17, 2024]

[222] Çelik B, Tomatsu SC, Tomatsu S, Khan SA. Epidemiology of mucopolysaccharidoses update. Diagnostics (Basel). 2021;**11**:273. DOI: 10.3390/diagnostics11020273 [Accessed: January 17, 2024]

[223] Kubaski F, de Oliveira Poswar F, Michelin-Tirelli K, Burin MG, Rojas-Málaga D, Brusius-Facchin A, et al. Diagnosis of mucopolysaccharidoses. Diagnostics (Basel). 2020;**10**:172. DOI: 10.3390/diagnostics10030172

[224] Brusius-Facchin AC, Siebert M, Leão D, Malaga DR, Pasqualim G, Trapp F, et al. Phenotype-oriented NGS panels for mucopolysaccharidoses: Validation and potential use in the diagnostic flowchart. Genetics and Molecular Biology. 2019;**42**:207-214. DOI: 10.1590/1678-4685-GMB-2018-0102 [Accessed: January 5, 2024]

[225] Hampe CS, Eisengart JB, Lund TC, Orchard PJ, Swietlicka M, Wesley J, et al. Mucopolysaccharidosis type I: A review of the natural history and molecular pathology. Cells (Basel, Switzerland). 2020;**9**:1838. DOI: 10.3390/cells9081838

[226] Clarke LA, Atherton AM, Burton BK, Day-Salvatore DL, Kaplan P, Leslie ND, et al. Mucopolysaccharidosis type I Newborn screening: Best practices for diagnosis and management. The Journal of Pediatrics. 2017;**182**:363-370. DOI: 10.1016/j.jpeds.2016.11.036 [Accessed: January 5, 2024]

[227] Nicolas-Jilwan M, AlSayed M. Mucopolysaccharidoses: Overview of neuroimaging manifestations. Pediatric Radiology. 2018;**48**:1503-1520. DOI: 10.1007/s00247-018-4139-3

[228] De Ponti G, Donsante S, Frigeni M, Pievani A, Corsi A, Bernardo ME, et al. MPSI manifestations and treatment outcome: Skeletal focus. International Journal of Molecular Sciences. 2022;**23**:11168. DOI: 10.3390/ijms231911168

[229] Clarke LA. Mucopolysaccharidosis Type I. Seattle, USA: GeneReviews®; 2024. Available from: https://www.ncbi.nlm.nih.gov/books/NBK1162/

[230] Clarke LA, Giugliani R, Guffon N, Jones SA, Keenan HA, Munoz-Rojas MV, et al. Genotype-phenotype relationships in mucopolysaccharidosis type I (MPS I): Insights from the International MPS I Registry. Clinical Genetics. 2019;**96**:281-289. DOI: 10.1111/cge.13583

[231] Pillai NR, Ahmed A, Vanyo T, Whitley CB. Early neonatal cardiac phenotype in hurler syndrome: Case report and literature review. Genes. 2022;**13**:1293. DOI: 10.3390/genes13081293

[232] Bie H, Yin J, He X, Kermode AR, Goddard-Borger E, Withers SG, et al. Insights into mucopolysaccharidosis I from the structure and action of

α-L-iduronidase. Nature Chemical Biology. 2013;**9**:739-745. DOI: 10.1038/nchembio.1357

[233] Peña-Gomar I, Jiménez-Mariscal JL, Cerón M, Rosas-Trigueros J, Reyes-López CA. c.1898C>G/p.Ser633Trp mutation in alpha-l-iduronidase: Clinical and structural implications. The Protein Journal. 2021;**40**:68-77. DOI: 10.1007/s10930-020-09950-9

[234] Li Y, Tang X, Meng Y, Luo G, Yu X. A novel compound mutation in alpha-L-iduronidase gene causes mucopolysaccharidosis type I. Journal of Genetics. 2019;**98**:1-4. DOI: 10.1007/s12041-019-1113-2

[235] Diogo R, Diogo L, Serra R, Almeida J, Oliveira A. Mucopolysaccharidosis type I: The importance of early diagnosis for adequate treatment. Curēus (Palo Alto, CA). 2023;**15**:e50595. DOI: 10.7759/cureus.50595

[236] Gardin A, Castelle M, Pichard S, Cano A, Chabrol B, Piarroux J, et al. Long term follow-up after haematopoietic stem cell transplantation for mucopolysaccharidosis type I-H: A retrospective study of 51 patients. Bone Marrow Transplantation (Basingstoke). 2023;**58**:295-302. DOI: 10.1038/s41409-022-01886-1

[237] Voskoboeva EY, Bookina TM, Semyachkina AN, Mikhaylova SV, Vashakmadze ND, Baydakova GV, et al. Mucopolysaccharidosis type I in the Russian Federation and Other Republics of the Former Soviet Union: Molecular genetic analysis and epidemiology. Frontiers in Molecular Biosciences. 2021;**8**:783644. DOI: 10.3389/fmolb.2021.783644 [Accessed: December 29, 2023]

[238] Yan L, Ding S, He Y, Fu B, Chen C, Li H. Whole paternal uniparental disomy of chromosome 4 with a novel homozygous IDUA splicing variant, c.159-9T>A, in a Chinese patient with mucopolysaccharidosis type I. Molecular Genetics & Genomic Medicine. 2024;**12**:e2507. DOI: 10.1002/mgg3.2507

[239] Asumda FZ, Kraker JA, Thomas SC, Maleszewski J, Stone EM, Lanpher BC, et al. Left-sided valvular heart disease and retinopathy in a 38-year-old woman with attenuated mucopolysaccharidosis: A case report. Therapeutic Advances in Rare Disease. 2023;**4**:263300402211459. DOI: 10.1177/26330040221145945

[240] Can NTB, Tran DM, Bui TP, Nguyen KN, Nguyen HH, Nguyen TV, et al. Molecular analysis of Vietnamese patients with mucopolysaccharidosis type I. Life (Basel). 2021;**11**:1162. DOI: 10.3390/life11111162 [Accessed: January 7, 2024]

[241] Zahoor MY, Cheema HA, Ijaz S, Anjum MN, Ramzan K, Bhinder MA. Mapping of IDUA gene variants in Pakistani patients with mucopolysaccharidosis type 1. Journal of Pediatric Endocrinology & Metabolism. 2019;**32**:1221-1227. DOI: 10.1515/jpem-2019-0188

[242] Adhikari AN, Gallagher RC, Wang Y, Currier RJ, Amatuni G, Bassaganyas L, et al. The role of exome sequencing in newborn screening for inborn errors of metabolism. Nature Medicine. 2020;**26**:1392-1397. DOI: 10.1038/s41591-020-0966-5

[243] Qian J, Wang X, Liu J, Zhong J, Le Y, Melchior Tellier LCA, et al. Applying targeted next generation sequencing to dried blood spot specimens from suspicious cases identified by tandem mass spectrometry-based newborn screening. Journal of Pediatric Endocrinology & Metabolism.

2017;**30**:979-988. DOI: 10.1515/jpem-2017-0003

[244] Kubaski F, Sousa I, Amorim T, Pereira D, Trometer J, Souza A, et al. Neonatal screening for MPS disorders in Latin America: A survey of pilot initiatives. International Journal of Neonatal Screening. 2020;**6**:90. DOI: 10.3390/ijns6040090

[245] Polo G, Gueraldi D, Giuliani A, Rubert L, Cazzorla C, Salviati L, et al. The combined use of enzyme activity and metabolite assays as a strategy for newborn screening of mucopolysaccharidosis type I. Clinical Chemistry and Laboratory Medicine. 2020;**58**:2063-2072. DOI: 10.1515/cclm-2020-0064

[246] Donati MA, Pasquini E, Spada M, Polo G, Burlina A. Newborn screening in mucopolysaccharidoses. Italian Journal of Pediatrics. 2018;**44**:126. DOI: 10.1186/s13052-018-0552-3 [Accessed: January 8, 2024]

[247] Gragnaniello V, Gueraldi D, Rubert L, Manzoni F, Cazzorla C, Giuliani A, et al. Report of five years of experience in neonatal screening for Mucopolysaccharidosis Type I and review of the literature. International Journal of Neonatal Screening. 2020;**6**:85. DOI: 10.3390/ijns6040085

[248] Jameson E, Jones S, Remmington T. Enzyme replacement therapy with laronidase (Aldurazyme(®)) for treating mucopolysaccharidosis type I. Cochrane Database of Systematic Reviews. 2016;**4**:CD009354. DOI: 10.1002/14651858.CD009354.pub4

[249] Hampe CS, Yund BD, Orchard PJ, Lund TC, Wesley J, McIvor RS. Differences in MPS I and MPS II disease manifestations. International Journal of Molecular Sciences. 2021;**22**:7888. DOI: 10.3390/ijms22157888

[250] D'Avanzo F, Rigon L, Zanetti A, Tomanin R. Mucopolysaccharidosis type II: One hundred years of research, diagnosis, and treatment. International Journal of Molecular Sciences. 2020;**21**:1258. DOI: 10.3390/ijms21041258

[251] Burton BK, Shively V, Quadri A, Warn L, Burton J, Grange DK, et al. Newborn screening for mucopolysaccharidosis type II: Lessons learned. Molecular Genetics and Metabolism. 2023;**140**:107557. DOI: 10.1016/j.ymgme.2023.107557

[252] Fukuhara Y, Miura A, Yamazaki N, So T, Kosuga M, Yanagi K, et al. A cDNA analysis disclosed the discordance of genotype-phenotype correlation in a patient with attenuated MPS II and a 76-base deletion in the gene for iduronate-2-sulfatase. Molecular Genetics and Metabolism Reports. 2020;**25**:100692. DOI: 10.1016/j.ymgmr.2020.100692

[253] Zhang W, Xie T, Sheng H, Shao Y, Lin Y, Jiang M, et al. Genetic analysis of 63 Chinese patients with mucopolysaccharidosis type II: Functional characterization of seven novel IDS variants. Clinica Chimica Acta. 2019;**491**:114-120. DOI: 10.1016/j.cca.2019.01.009

[254] Jezela-Stanek A, Pokora P, Młynek M, Smyk M, Ziemkiewicz K,Różdżyńska-Świątkowska A, et al. Diverse clinical outcome of Hunter syndrome in patients with chromosomal aberration encompassing entire and partial IDS deletions: What is important for early diagnosis and counseling? Clinical Dysmorphology. 2021;**30**:76-82. DOI: 10.1097/MCD.0000000000000344

[255] Wei X, Jin F, Ye Y, Xu C, Qu N, Ju X, et al. A novel mutation of IDS gene in a Chinese patient with mucopolysaccharidosis II by

next-generation sequencing. Clinica Chimica Acta. 2011;**412**:2340-2342. DOI: 10.1016/j.cca.2011.08.031 [Accessed: January 9, 2024]

[256] Tang J, Chang G, Wei M, Li X, Chen H, Qin Y, et al. Diagnosis of patients with mucopolysaccharidosis type II via RNA sequencing. Clinica Chimica Acta. 2022;**537**:38-45. DOI: 10.1016/j.cca.2022.10.007

[257] Semyachkina AN, Voskoboeva EY, Zakharova EY, Nikolaeva EA, Kanivets IV, Kolotii AD, et al. Case report: A rare case of Hunter syndrome (type II mucopolysaccharidosis) in a girl. BMC Medical Genetics. 2019;**20**:66. DOI: 10.1186/s12881-019-0807-x

[258] Oliveira Netto AB, Brusius-Facchin A, Leistner-Segal S, Kubaski F, Josahkian J, Giugliani R. Detection of mosaic variants in mothers of MPS II patients by next generation sequencing. Frontiers in Molecular Biosciences. 2021;**8**:789350. DOI: 10.3389/fmolb.2021.789350

[259] Yee KS, Alexanderian D, Martin S, Olayinka-Amao B, Whiteman DAH. Clinical investigator perspectives on patient outcomes in children with neuronopathic mucopolysaccharidosis II during intrathecal idursulfase-IT treatment. Orphanet Journal of Rare Diseases. 2024;**19**:158. DOI: 10.1186/s13023-024-03147-4

[260] Ream MA, Lam WKK, Grosse SD, Ojodu J, Jones E, Prosser LA, et al. Evidence and recommendation for mucopolysaccharidosis type II newborn screening in the United States. Genetics in Medicine. 2024;**25**(2):100330. DOI: 10.1016/j.gim.2022.10.012

[261] Almenabawy N, Ramadan M, Kamel M, Mahmoud IG, Amer F, Shaheen Y, et al. Clinical, biochemical, and molecular characterization of mucopolysaccharidosis type III in 34 Egyptian patients. American Journal of Medical Genetics. Part A. 2023;**191**:2354-2363. DOI: 10.1002/ajmg.a.63342

[262] Lin H, Chuang C, Lee C, Tu R, Lo Y, Chiu PC, et al. Mucopolysaccharidosis III in Taiwan: Natural history, clinical and molecular characteristics of 28 patients diagnosed during a 21-year period. American Journal of Medical Genetics. Part A. 2018;**176**:1799-1809. DOI: 10.1002/ajmg.a.40351

[263] Kong W, Meng Y, Zou L, Yang G, Wang J, Shi X. Mucopolysaccharidosis III in Mainland China: Natural history, clinical and molecular characteristics of 34 patients. Journal of Pediatric Endocrinology & Metabolism. 2020;**33**:793-802. DOI: 10.1515/jpem-2019-0505

[264] Kim M, Yang A, Noh E, Kim C, Bae GY, Lim HH, et al. Natural history and molecular characteristics of Korean patients with mucopolysaccharidosis type III. Journal of Personalized Medicine. 2022;**12**:665. DOI: 10.3390/jpm12050665

[265] Gul R, Firasat S, Schubert M, Ullah A, Peña E, Thuesen ACB, et al. Identification of genetic variants associated with a wide spectrum of phenotypes clinically diagnosed as Sanfilippo and Morquio syndromes using whole genome sequencing. Frontiers in Genetics. 2023;**14**:1254909. DOI: 10.3389/fgene.2023.1254909

[266] Alyazidi AS, Muthaffar OY, Baaishrah LS, Shawli MK, Jambi AT, Aljezani MA, et al. Current concepts in the Management of Sanfilippo Syndrome (MPS III): A narrative review. Curēus (Palo Alto, CA). 2024;**16**:e58023. DOI: 10.7759/cureus.58023

[267] Seker Yilmaz B, Davison J, Jones SA, Baruteau J. Novel therapies for mucopolysaccharidosis type III. Journal of Inherited Metabolic Disease. 2021;**44**:129-147. DOI: 10.1002/jimd.12316

[268] Li X, Xiao R, Chen B, Yang G, Zhang X, Fu Z, et al. A novel mutation of SGSH and clinical features analysis of mucopolysaccharidosis type IIIA. Medicine (Baltimore). 2018;**97**:1-6. DOI: 10.1097/md.0000000000013758

[269] Sansović I, Odak L, Bobinec A, Barišić I. 97 A novel missense mutation in SGSH gene causing Sanfillipo type 3A mucopolysaccharidosis. Archives of Disease in Childhood. 2021;**106**:A41. DOI: 10.1136/archdischild-2021-europaediatrics.97

[270] De Falco A, Karali M, Criscuolo C, Testa F, Barillari MR, Scarpato M, et al. Late-onset mucopolysaccharidosis type IIIA mimicking usher syndrome. American Journal of Medical Genetics. Part A. 2024;**194**:e63517. DOI: 10.1002/ajmg.a.63517

[271] Zabihi R, Zamani M, Aminzadeh M, Chamanrou N, Kiani FZ, Seifi T, et al. Identification of new variants in patients with mucopolysaccharidosis in consanguineous Iranian families. Frontiers in Genetics. 2024;**15**:1343094. DOI: 10.3389/fgene.2024.1343094

[272] Rey LM, Sánchez TA, Naranjo DC, Cuesta HV. A novel mutation (p.Met1?) of a Cuban patient in the NAGLU gene with mucopolysaccharidosis IIIB. Journal of Inborn Errors of Metabolism and Screening. 2021;**9**:1-5. DOI:10.1590/2326-4594-jiems-2021-0013

[273] Selmer KK, Gilfillan GD, Munthe LA, Braekken SK, Undlien DE, Strømme P, et al. A mild form of mucopolysaccharidosis IIIB diagnosed with targeted next-generation sequencing of linked genomic regions. European Journal of Human Genetics: EJHG. 2012;**20**:58-63. DOI: 10.1038/ejhg.2011.126

[274] Zeng Q, Fan Y, Wang L, Huang Z, Gu X, Yu Y. Molecular defects identified by whole exome sequencing in a child with atypical mucopolysaccharidosis IIIB. Journal of Pediatric Endocrinology & Metabolism. 2017;**30**:463-469. DOI: 10.1515/jpem-2016-0333

[275] Ozkinay F, Emecen DA, Kose M, Isik E, Bozaci AE, Canda E, et al. Clinical and genetic features of 13 patients with mucopolysaccarhidosis type IIIB: Description of two novel NAGLU gene mutations. Molecular Genetics and Metabolism Reports. 2021;**27**:1-5. DOI: 10.1016/j.ymgmr.2021.100732

[276] Khorrami M, Mahdavi M, Fakhr F, Kheirollahi M. A novel pathogenic variant in NAGLU (N-acetyl-alpha-glucosaminidase) gene identified by targeted next-generation sequencing followed by in silico analysis. Iranian Journal of Child Neurology. 2019;**13**:173-183. DOI: 10.22037/ijcn.v13i4.19894

[277] Li J, Xie H, Jiang Y. Mucopolysaccharidosis IIIB and mild skeletal anomalies: Coexistence of NAGLU and CYP26B1 missense variations in the same patient in a Chinese family. BMC Medical Genetics. 2018;**19**:51. DOI: 10.1186/s12881-018-0562-4

[278] Alaei MR, Kheirkhahan M, Talebi S, Davoudi-Dehaghani E, Keramatipour M. Once in a blue moon, a very rare coexistence of glutaric acidemia type I and mucopolysaccharidosis type IIIB in a patient. Iranian Biomedical Journal. 2020;**24**:201-205. DOI: 10.29252/ibj.24.3.201

[279] Muschol N, Giugliani R, Jones SA, Muenzer J, Smith NJC, Whitley CB, et al. Sanfilippo syndrome: Consensus guidelines for clinical care. Orphanet Journal of Rare Diseases. 2022;**17**:1-391. DOI: 10.1186/s13023-022-02484-6

[280] Zhao B, Cao Z, Zheng Y, Nguyen P, Bowen A, Edwards RH, et al. Structural and mechanistic insights into a lysosomal membrane enzyme HGSNAT involved in Sanfilippo syndrome. Nature Communications. 2024;**15**:5388-5310. DOI: 10.1038/s41467-024-49614-1

[281] Taherzadeh M, Zhang E, Londono I, De Leener B, Wang S, Cooper JD, et al. Severe central nervous system demyelination in Sanfilippo disease. Frontiers in Molecular Neuroscience. 2023;**16**:1323449. DOI: 10.3389/fnmol.2023.1323449

[282] Martins C, Frassinetti V de Medeiros P, Leistner-Segal S, Dridi L, Elcioglu N. et al. Molecular characterization of a large group of mucopolysaccharidosis type IIIC patients reveals the evolutionary history of the disease. Human Mutations. 2019;**40**(8)1084-1100. DOI: 10.1002/humu.23752

[283] Liang Y, Gao X, Lu D, Zhang H, Zhang. Mucopolysaccharidosis type IIIC in Chinese mainland: Clinical and molecular characteristics of ten patients and report of six novel variants in the HGSNAT gene. Metabolic Brain Disease. 2023;**38**:2013-2023. DOI: 10.1007/s11011-023-01204-8

[284] Zhao H, Wang L, Zhang M, Wang H, Zhang S, Wu J, et al. Identification and characterization of novel genetic variants in the first Chinese family of mucopolysaccharidosis IIIC (Sanfilippo C syndrome). Journal of Cellular and Molecular Medicine. 2024;**28**:e18307. DOI: 10.1111/jcmm.18307

[285] Schiff ER, Daich Varela M, Robson AG, Pierpoint K, Ba-Abbad R, Nutan S, et al. A genetic and clinical study of individuals with nonsyndromic retinopathy consequent upon sequence variants in HGSNAT, the gene associated with Sanfilippo C mucopolysaccharidosis. American Journal of Medical Genetics. Part C, Seminars in Medical Genetics. 2020;**184**:631-643. DOI: 10.1002/ajmg.c.31822

[286] Ludwig J, Sawant OB, Wood J, Singamsetty S, Pan X, Bonilha VL, et al. Histological characterization of retinal degeneration in mucopolysaccharidosis type IIIC. Experimental Eye Research. 2023;**229**:109433. DOI: 10.1016/j.exer.2023.109433

[287] Carrera W, Ng C, Burckhard B, Ng J, McDonald HR, Agarwal A. Nonsyndromic retinitis pigmentosa with bilateral retinal neovascularization due to Hgsnat mutation. Retinal Cases & Brief Reports. 2023;**17**:348-351. DOI: 10.1097/ICB.0000000000001193

[288] Haer-Wigman L, Newman H, Leibu R, Bax NM, Baris HN, Rizel L, et al. Non-syndromic retinitis pigmentosa due to mutations in the mucopolysaccharidosis type IIIC Gene, heparan-alpha-glucosaminide N-acetyltransferase (HGSNAT). Human Molecular Genetics. 2015;**24**:3742-3751. DOI: 10.1093/hmg/ddv118

[289] da Palma MM, Marra M, Igelman AD, Ku CA, Burr A, Andersen K, et al. Expanding the phenotypic and genotypic spectrum of patients with HGSNAT-related retinopathy. Ophthalmic Genetics. 2024;**45**:167-174. DOI: 10.1080/13816810.2023.2245035

[290] Minami K, Morimoto H, Morioka H, Imakiire A, Kinoshita M, Yamamoto R, et al. Pathogenic roles

of Heparan sulfate and its use as a biomarker in mucopolysaccharidoses. International Journal of Molecular Sciences. 2022;**23**:11724. DOI: 10.3390/ijms231911724

[291] Santhoshkumar R, Mahale RR, Kishore PK, Chickabasaviah YT. Child neurology: Mucopolysaccharidosis IIID: Evidence from ultrastructural and genomic study. Neurology. 2023;**101**:e1572-e1576. DOI: 10.1212/WNL.0000000000207647

[292] Beesley CE, Concolino D, Filocamo M, Winchester BG, Strisciuglio P. Identification and characterisation of an 8.7kb deletion and a novel nonsense mutation in two Italian families with Sanfilippo syndrome type D (mucopolysaccharidosis IIID). Molecular Genetics and Metabolism. 2007;**90**:77-80. DOI: 10.1016/j.ymgme.2006.07.014

[293] Wang F, Moen DR, Sauni C, Kan S, Li S, Le SQ, et al. Enzyme replacement therapy for mucopolysaccharidosis IIID using recombinant human α-N-acetylglucosamine-6-sulfatase in neonatal mice. Molecular Pharmaceutics. 2021;**18**:214-227. DOI: 10.1021/acs.molpharmaceut.0c00831

[294] Liu Y, Gelb MH. Tandem mass spectrometric assay of N-acetylglucosamine-6-sulfatase for multiplex analysis of mucopolysaccharidosis-IIID in dried blood spots. Molecular Genetics and Metabolism. 2024;**141**:108105. DOI: 10.1016/j.ymgme.2023.108105

[295] McBride KL, Flanigan KM. Update in the mucopolysaccharidoses. Seminars in Pediatric Neurology. 2021;**37**:100874. DOI: 10.1016/j.spen.2021.100874

[296] Tüysüz B, Alkaya DU, Toksoy G, Güneş N, Yıldırım T, Bayhan İA, et al. Mutation spectrum and pivotal features for differential diagnosis of mucopolysaccharidosis IVA patients with severe and attenuated phenotype. Gene. 2019;**704**:59-67. DOI: 10.1016/j.gene.2019.04.026

[297] Zanetti A, D'Avanzo F, AlSayed M, Brusius-Facchin AC, Chien Y, Giugliani R, et al. Molecular basis of mucopolysaccharidosis IVA (Morquio A syndrome): A review and classification of GALNS gene variants and reporting of 68 novel variants. Human Mutation. 2021;**42**:1384-1398. DOI: 10.1002/humu.24270

[298] Xie J, Pan J, Guo D, Pan W, Li R, Guo C, et al. Mutation analysis and pathogenicity identification of mucopolysaccharidosis type IVA in 8 South China families. Gene. 2019;**686**:261-269. DOI: 10.1016/j.gene.2018.11.051

[299] Yi M, Shen P, Zhang H. Delayed diagnosis of mild mucopolysaccharidosis type IVA. BMC Medical Genomics. 2024;**17**:1-151. DOI: 10.1186/s12920-024-01910-x

[300] Cárdenas JM, Vergara D, Witting S, Balut F, Guerra P, Mesa JT, et al. Genotype and phenotype characterization of patients with mucopolysaccharidosis IV-A in Chile. Molecular Syndromology. 2023;**14**:416-427. DOI: 10.1159/000529807

[301] Caciotti A, Tonin R, Mort M, Cooper DN, Gasperini S, Rigoldi M, et al. Mis-splicing of the GALNS gene resulting from deep intronic mutations as a cause of Morquio a disease. BMC Medical Genetics. 2018;**19**:183. DOI: 10.1186/s12881-018-0694-6

[302] Pachajoa H, Amparo Acosta M, Alméciga-Díaz CJ, Ariza Y, et al. Molecular characterization of mucopolysaccharidosis type IVA

patients in the Andean region of Colombia. American Journal of Medical Genetics Part C: Seminars in Medical Genetics. 2021;**187**(3):388-395. DOI: 10.1002/ajmg.c.31936

[303] Tebani A, Sudrié-Arnaud B, Dabaj I, Torre S, Domitille L, Snanoudj S, et al. Disentangling molecular and clinical stratification patterns in beta-galactosidase deficiency. Journal of Medical Genetics. 2022;**59**:377-384. DOI: 10.1136/jmedgenet-2020-107510

[304] Pedersen JJ, Duno M, Wibrand F, Hammer C, Krag T, Vissing J. β-Galactosidase deficiency in the GLB1 spectrum of lysosomal storage disease can present with severe muscle weakness and atrophy. JIMD Reports. 2022;**63**:540-545. DOI: 10.1002/jmd2.12324

[305] Abumansour IS, Yuskiv N, Paschke E, Stockler-Ipsiroglu S. Morquio-B disease: Clinical and genetic characteristics of a distinct *GLB1*-related dysostosis multiplex. JIMD Reports. 2020;**51**:30-44. DOI: 10.1002/jmd2.12065

[306] Lawrence R, Van Vleet JL, Mangini L, Harris A, Martin N, Clark W, et al. Characterization of glycan substrates accumulating in GM1 gangliosidosis. Molecular Genetics and Metabolism Reports. 2019;**21**:100524. DOI: 10.1016/j.ymgmr.2019.100524

[307] Caciotti A, Cellai L, Tonin R, Mei D, Procopio E, Di Rocco M, et al. Morquio B disease: From pathophysiology towards diagnosis. Molecular Genetics and Metabolism. 2021;**132**:180-188. DOI: 10.1016/j.ymgme.2021.01.008

[308] Stockler-Ipsiroglu S, Yazdanpanah N, Yazdanpanah M, Moisa Popurs M, Yuskiv N, Schmitz Ferreira Santos ML, et al. Morquio-like dysostosis multiplex presenting with neuronopathic features is a distinct GLB1-related phenotype. JIMD Reports. 2021;**60**:23-31. DOI: 10.1002/jmd2.12211

[309] Gholamian T, Chhina H, Stockler S, Cooper A. Morquio B disease: A case report. Frontiers in Pediatrics. 2024;**12**:1285414. DOI: 10.3389/fped.2024.1285414

[310] Yuskiv N, Higaki K, Stockler-Ipsiroglu S. Morquio B disease. Disease characteristics and treatment options of a distinct GLB1-related dysostosis multiplex. International Journal of Molecular Sciences. 2020;**21**:9121. DOI: 10.3390/ijms21239121

[311] D'Avanzo F, Zanetti A, De Filippis C, Tomanin R. Mucopolysaccharidosis type VI, an updated overview of the disease. International Journal of Molecular Sciences. 2021;**22**:13456. DOI: 10.3390/ijms222413456

[312] Jafaryazdi R, Shams S, Isaian A, Setoodeh A, Teimourian S. Identification of eleven different mutations including six novel, in the arylsulfatase B gene in Iranian patients with mucopolysaccharidosis type VI. Molecular Biology Reports. 2019;**46**:3417-3426. DOI: 10.1007/s11033-019-04804-9

[313] Aminzadeh M, Malekpour N, Ghandil P. Identification of arylsulfatase B gene mutations and clinical presentations of Iranian patients with mucopolysaccharidosis VI. Gene. 2019;**706**:1-5. DOI: 10.1016/j.gene.2019.04.050

[314] Voskoboeva E, Semyachkina A, Miklyaev O, Gamzatova A, Mikhaylova S, Vashakmadze N, et al. Epidemiology and genetics of mucopolysaccharidosis type VI in Russia. Frontiers in Molecular Biosciences. 2022;**8**:780184. DOI: 10.3389/fmolb.2021.780184

[315] Malekpour N, Vakili R, Hamzehloie T. Mutational analysis of ARSB gene in mucopolysaccharidosis type VI: Identification of three novel mutations in Iranian patients. Iranian Journal of Basic Medical Sciences. 2018;**21**:950-956. DOI: 10.22038/IJBMS.2018.27742.6760

[316] Marek-Yagel D, Eliyahu A, Veber A, Shalva N, Philosoph AM, Barel O, et al. Deep intronic variant in the ARSB gene as the genetic cause for Maroteaux–Lamy syndrome (MPS VI). American Journal of Medical Genetics. Part A. 2021;**185**:3804-3809. DOI: 10.1002/ajmg.a.62453

[317] He M, Yang J, Dong M, Wang Y, Liu H. Compound heterozygous missense mutations in a Chinese mucopolysaccharidosis type VI patient: A case report. BMC Ophthalmology. 2021;**21**:214. DOI: 10.1186/s12886-021-01979-3

[318] Tomanin R, Karageorgos L, Zanetti A, Al-Sayed M, Bailey M, Miller N, et al. Mucopolysaccharidosis type VI (MPS VI) and molecular analysis: Review and classification of published variants in the ARSB gene. Human Mutation. 2018;**39**:1788-1802. DOI: 10.1002/humu.23613

[319] Akyol MU, Alden TD, Amartino H, Ashworth J, Belani K, Berger KI, et al. Recommendations for the management of MPS VI: Systematic evidence- and consensus-based guidance. Orphanet Journal of Rare Diseases. 2019;**14**:118. DOI: 10.1186/s13023-019-1080-y

[320] Khan FI, Shahbaaz M, Bisetty K, Waheed A, Sly WS, Ahmad F, et al. Large scale analysis of the mutational landscape in β-glucuronidase: A major player of mucopolysaccharidosis type VII. Gene. 2016;**576**:36-44. DOI: 10.1016/j.gene.2015.09.062

[321] Grant CL, López-Valdez J, Marsden D, Ezgü F. Mucopolysaccharidosis type VII (sly syndrome) - What do we know? Molecular Genetics and Metabolism. 2024;**141**:108145. DOI: 10.1016/j.ymgme.2024.108145

[322] Poyatos-Andújar AM, García-Linares S, Carretero P, Ocon O, Fresneda D, Gort L, et al. Prenatal mucopolysaccharidosis VII: A novel pathogenic variant identified in GUSB gene. Clinical Case Reports. 2021;**9**:790-795. DOI: 10.1002/ccr3.3644

[323] Du R, Tian H, Zhao B, Shi X, Sun Y, Qiu B, et al. A de novo homozygous missense mutation of the GUSB gene leads to mucopolysaccharidosis type VII identification in a family with twice adverse pregnancy outcomes due to non-immune hydrops fetalis. Molecular Genetics and Metabolism Reports. 2024;**38**:101033. DOI: 10.1016/j.ymgmr.2023.101033

[324] Montaño AM, Lock-Hock N, Steiner RD, Graham BH, Szlago M, Greenstein R, et al. Clinical course of sly syndrome (mucopolysaccharidosis type VII). Journal of Medical Genetics. 2016;**53**:403-418. DOI: 10.1136/jmedgenet-2015-103322

[325] Gónzalez-Meneses A, Pineda M, Bandeira A, Janeiro P, Ruiz MÃ, Diogo L, et al. Description of the molecular and clinical characteristics of the mucopolysaccharidosis type VII Iberian cohort. Orphanet Journal of Rare Diseases. 2021;**16**:1-445. DOI: 10.1186/s13023-021-02063-1

[326] Guffon N, Froissart R, Fouilhoux A. A rare late progression form of sly syndrome mucopolysaccharidosis. JIMD Reports. 2019;**49**:1-6. DOI: 10.1002/jmd2.12039

[327] Yang C, Pan J, Linpeng S, Li Z, Tan H, Wu L. Identification of five novel

mutations causing rare lysosomal storage diseases. Medical Science Monitor. 2019;**25**:7634-7644. DOI: 10.12659/MSM.915876

[328] Lee C, Chuang C, Hsu C, Chiu H, Tu R, Lo Y, et al. The first mucopolysaccharidosis type VII in a Taiwanese girl: A case report and review of the literature. Journal of the Formosan Medical Association. 2022;**121**:712-717. DOI: 10.1016/j.jfma.2021.07.024

[329] Dubot P, Sabourdy F, Plat G, Jubert C, Cancès C, Broué P, et al. First report of a patient with MPS type VII, due to novel mutations in GUSB, who underwent enzyme replacement and then hematopoietic stem cell transplantation. International Journal of Molecular Sciences. 2019;**20**:5345. DOI: 10.3390/ijms20215345

[330] Tomatsu S, Orii KO, Islam MR, Shah GN, Grubb JH, Sukegawa K, et al. Methylation patterns of the human β-glucuronidase gene locus: Boundaries of methylation and general implications for frequent point mutations at CpG dinucleotides. Genomics (San Diego, California). 2002;**79**:363-375. DOI: 10.1006/geno.2002.6706

[331] Poswar FDO, Henriques Nehm J, Kubaski F, Poletto E, Giugliani R. Diagnosis and emerging treatment strategies for mucopolysaccharidosis VII (sly syndrome). Therapeutics and Clinical Risk Management. 2022;**18**:1143-1155. DOI: 10.2147/TCRM.S351300

[332] Giugliani R, Barth AL, Dumas MRC, da Silva Franco JF, de Rosso Giuliani L, Grangeiro CHP, et al. Mucopolysaccharidosis VII in Brazil: Natural history and clinical findings. Orphanet Journal of Rare Diseases. 2021;**16**:1-238. DOI: 10.1186/s13023-021-01870-w

[333] Chandler NJ, Ramachandran V, Beesley C, Otigbah C, Davison J, Ashraf T. Prenatal diagnosis of mucopolysaccharidosis type VII facilitating treatment in neonatal period. Prenatal Diagnosis. 2023;**43**:1567-1569. DOI: 10.1002/pd.6455

[334] Giugliani R, Gonzalez-Meneses A, Scarpa M, Burton B, Wang R, Martins E, et al. Disease characteristics, effectiveness, and safety of vestronidase alfa for the treatment of patients with mucopolysaccharidosis VII in a novel, longitudinal, multicenter disease monitoring program. Orphanet Journal of Rare Diseases. 2024;**19**:189. DOI: 10.1186/s13023-024-03176-z

[335] Fink SP, Triggs-Raine B. Genetic deficiencies of hyaluronan degradation. Cells (Basel, Switzerland). 2024;**13**:1203. DOI: 10.3390/cells13141203

[336] Preston CG, Wright MW, Madhavrao R, Harrison SM, Goldstein JL, Luo X, et al. ClinGen variant curation Interface: A variant classification platform for the application of evidence criteria from ACMG/AMP guidelines. Genome Medicine. 2022;**14**:6. DOI: 10.1186/s13073-021-01004-8

[337] Verheyen S, Blatterer J, Speicher MR, Bhavani GS, Boons G, Ilse M, et al. Novel subtype of mucopolysaccharidosis caused by arylsulfatase K (ARSK) deficiency. Journal of Medical Genetics. 2022;**59**:957-964. DOI: 10.1136/jmedgenet-2021-108061

[338] Sofronova V, Gotovtseva L, Danilova A, Sukhomyasova A, Moriwaki T, Terawaki S, et al. Prenatal diagnosis of Mucopolysaccharidosis-plus syndrome (MPSPS). Genes. 2023;**14**:1581. DOI: 10.3390/genes14081581

[339] Kingsmore SF. Dispatches from Biotech beginning BeginNGS: Rapid

newborn genome sequencing to end the diagnostic and therapeutic odyssey. American Journal of Medical Genetics. Part C, Seminars in Medical Genetics. 2022;**190**:243-256. DOI: 10.1002/ajmg.c.32005

[340] Might M, Crouse AB. Why rare disease needs precision medicine—And precision medicine needs rare disease. Cell Reports. Medicine. 2022;**3**:100530. DOI: 10.1016/j.xcrm.2022.100530

[341] Encarnação M, Coutinho MF, Silva L, Ribeiro D, Ouesleti S, Campos T, et al. Assessing lysosomal disorders in the NGS era: Identification of novel rare variants. International Journal of Molecular Sciences. 2020;**21**:6355. DOI: 10.3390/ijms21176355 [Accessed: January 19, 2024]

[342] Marshall CR, Chowdhury S, Taft RJ, Lebo MS, Buchan JG, Harrison SM, et al. Best practices for the analytical validation of clinical whole-genome sequencing intended for the diagnosis of germline disease. NPJ Genomic Medicine. 2020;**5**:47. DOI: 10.1038/s41525-020-00154-9

[343] U.S. Department of Health and Human Services. Considerations for design, development, and analytical validation of next generation sequencing-based in vitro diagnostics intended to aid in the diagnosis of suspected germline diseases. In: Guidance for Stakeholders and Food and Drug Administration Staff. Vol. 83. The Federal Register; 2018. p. 16106

[344] Sarata AK. Regulation of Laboratory-Developed Tests : FDA's Proposed Rule / Amanda K. Sarata: CRS Reports (Library of Congress Congressional Research Service); 2024

[345] Sarata AK. Congressional Research Service Issues in focus White Paper on Regulation of Laboratory-Developed Tests - FDA's Proposed Rule. Targeted News Service; 2024

[346] Lurie P. Center for Science in the Public Interest: FDA Finalizes Much-Needed Rule to Regulate Laboratory-Developed Tests. Targeted News Service; 2024

[347] Groopman E, Fernandez R, Mohan S, Stafford A, Weaver M, Clarke L, et al. The ClinGen lysosomal diseases gene curation panel: Applying a standardized curation framework to assess the clinical validity of genes for lysosomal disease. Molecular Genetics and Metabolism. 2023;**138**:107128. DOI: 10.1016/j.ymgme.2022.107128

[348] Milko LV, Funke BH, Hershberger RE, Azzariti DR, Lee K, Riggs ER, et al. Development of clinical domain working groups for the clinical genome resource (ClinGen): Lessons learned and plans for the future. Genetics in Medicine. 2019;**21**:987-993. DOI: 10.1038/s41436-018-0267-2

[349] Jalal K, Carter RL, Barczykowski A, Tomatsu S, Langan TJ. A roadmap for potential improvement of newborn screening for inherited metabolic diseases following recent developments and successful applications of bivariate normal limits for pre-symptomatic detection of MPS I, Pompe disease, and Krabbe disease. International Journal of Neonatal Screening. 2022;**8**:61. DOI: 10.3390/ijns8040061

[350] Reyhani-Ardabili M, Ghafouri-Fard S. CRISPR/Cas9 technology in the modeling of and treatment of mucopolysaccharidosis. Biochemistry and Biophysics Reports. 2024;**39**:101771. DOI: 10.1016/j.bbrep.2024.101771

Chapter 5

Prevention of Neurological Sequels in Infants with Perinatal Brain Damage Using Katona's Neurohabilitation Procedure

Thalía Harmony

Abstract

We aim to describe evaluations and early treatments to prevent neurological sequels in the outcome. Preterm and term infants with prenatal and perinatal risk factors for perinatal brain damage were studied. MRI examinations showed that 80% of these infants with risk factors have abnormal structural brain findings suggesting brain damage. This fact suggested that they must be treated as soon as possible. Katona's neurohabilitation procedure was described, and the results obtained with different samples of term and preterm infants showed that its application prevented neurologic sequels. The outcome for the infants between 70 and 80% was favorable. The conclusion was that infants with prenatal and perinatal risk factors for brain damage should be treated immediately.

Keywords: perinatal brain damage, prenatal risk factors, perinatal risk factors, MRI, Katona's therapy

1. Introduction

Perinatal brain damage (PBD) is a term used for brain lesions observed in term and preterm newborns. The main pathologies are hypoxic-ischemic encephalopathy (HIE) and encephalopathy of prematurity (EOP). The effects of these pathologies on the brain are very different and characterized by neurological sequels, such as cerebral palsy (CP) and other motor insufficiencies, sensorial (blindness, deafness), perceptual and cognitive problems (intellectual retardation, learning difficulties, and attention problems), and adverse neuropsychiatric development [1]. The most severe sequel is CP, characterized by motor and mental deficiencies. However, there are other motor sequels, such as deficits in coordination and minor motor difficulties. The most frequent cognitive deficit is attention deficit hyperactivity disorder (ADHD).

Evidence suggests that brain development may be particularly vulnerable to factors such as maternal nutrition, infection, and stress during pregnancy. This review discusses how maternal factors can affect brain development and outcomes in offspring.

The literature states that perinatal brain lesions and neurodevelopment problems are frequently due to prenatal and perinatal risk factors [2, 3]. Chorioamnionitis has been associated with a higher risk for hypoxic-ischemic encephalopathy (HIE) and cerebral palsy (CP) in both preterm and term-born neonates. In addition, maternal stress and inflammation during any trimester, in the absence of direct fetal brain infection, can negatively affect neurodevelopmental outcomes [4].

Unfortunately, these antecedents in the presence of apparently "normal" newborns are often dismissed in the newborn period and not considered for a follow-up of the child. This occurs in many undeveloped countries or some populations of rich countries. Late clinical observations by parents or medical professionals, as delays in developmental milestones, are the first elements to diagnose the brain lesion. It is too late to make use of brain plasticity. Brain plasticity decreases after the newborn period, while the brain lesions are not yet clinically expressed (See **Figure 1**).

Therefore, there is a period when brain plasticity is high, and the lesion has not been expressed to begin the therapy. This period is used in Katona's therapy [5].

To dismiss the presence of antecedents of risk factors and begin therapy once the lesion is clinically expressed (delayed presence of developmental milestones) are one of the causes of the high rate of neurologic disabilities due to these factors. A report on the global prevalence of disabilities among children and adolescents [6] born before 33 weeks of gestation indicates that 291.3 million (11.3%) children younger than 20 years have mild-to-severe disabilities, according to [7].

Perinatal brain injury affects infants born at all gestational ages, but its incidence and morbidity increase with decreasing gestational age [8–10]. In another meta-analysis, preterm infants were found at an increased risk for language, cognitive, sensory, and motor deficits [11]. Other causes of brain traumas are due to improper obstetric instrumental techniques such as forceps delivery and vacuum extraction. These procedures increase the ease of the descendant baby during labor but may produce brain injuries [12, 13]. These obstetric errors may be attributable to poor health services and lack of mothers' education.

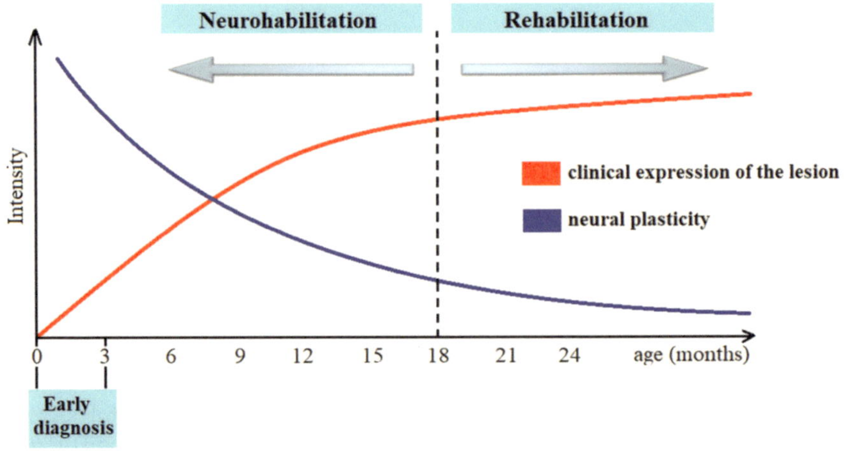

Figure 1.
This figure shows the trend of brain plasticity (red line) and the clinical expression of the lesion (blue line). The x-axis shows the infant's age in months, and the y-axis shows the intensity of these processes. During the first three months, the diagnosis or findings of antecedents of prenatal or perinatal risk factors for brain damage should be made. Katona's neurohabilitation therapy should begin, which ends when the infant's independent walking is reached.

1.1 Prenatal and perinatal risk factors

In recent years, the survival of preterm newborns has increased due to advanced medical procedures; however, this has resulted in a rising number of infants with long-term developmental problems. Preterm infants are at considerably increased risk of mortality as well as respiratory and non-respiratory morbidity. Equally, there is evidence that these infants may be at increased risk of long-term neurocognitive and behavioral problems and reduced school performance [14].

In a recent review by [4], acquired brain injuries during the different trimesters of pregnancy and in the postnatal brain are referred to. White matter injury and germinal matrix hemorrhage/intraventricular hemorrhage in preterm infants and hypoxic-ischemic encephalopathy in term infants are the main pathologies studied by these authors. During the first trimester, it is very important to ensure maternal health. Infections may affect the placenta and fetal neurodevelopment, producing neural tube defects in 0.74 per 1000 births. Folate deficiency is the main nutritional risk factor for neural tube defects, which can be prevented by prenatal folate intake. During the second trimester, the cerebral cortex is formed, and insults such as maternal alcohol use, tobacco, or other drugs of abuse in utero may produce cortical structural alterations. These facts may also alter the development of the corpus callosum. In the third trimester, myelination, synaptogenesis, and axonal pruning begin. Fetal brain infarcts or hemorrhages produce severe structural defects. Maternal infections can lead to neonatal encephalopathy [4].

Prolonged labor lasting more than 20 hours for the first delivery and more than 14 hours in those who have previously given birth, fetal distress, and perinatal asphyxia are other factors that may produce fetal brain deficiencies. Congenital neural tube anomalies are also due to multifactorial causes, including prenatal and perinatal risk factors [15]. Other important prenatal and perinatal risk factors for perinatal brain damage are the mother's age, previous abortions, toxemia, growth restriction in utero, lower weight at birth for the gestational age, congenital heart anomalies, anemia, necrotizing enterocolitis, and respiratory distress [16].

Lower Apgar Score (<7) affects neurodevelopment in infants born small for gestational age [17], and it is used routinely to detect problems in newborns.

In 2017, [18] published a Table of prenatal and perinatal risk factors in 262 infants from 25 to 40 weeks of gestational age (WGA). In the groups of 25 to 27 and 28 to 29 WGA, the most frequent factors were sepsis, asphyxia, and very low weight at birth (VLW). From 30 to 31 WGA, toxemia, VLW, and metabolic problems were the most frequent. Maternal infections, VLW, asphyxia, and sepsis were frequently observed between 32 and 34 WGA. At term, maternal infections and asphyxia were the most frequent risk factors.

We may conclude that following mothers during gestation and newborns during labor is very important. Now, according to [19], "pregnancy-related deaths and diseases remain unacceptably high. In 2015, an estimated 303,000 women died from pregnancy-related causes, 2.7 million babies died during the first 28 days of life, and 2.6 million babies were stillborn. While substantial progress has been made over the past two decades, increased access to, and use of, higher-quality health care during pregnancy and childbirth can prevent many of these deaths and diseases, as well as improve women and adolescent girls' experience of pregnancy and childbirth. Globally, however, only 64% of women receive antenatal care four or more times throughout their pregnancy".

1.2 MRI findings

The term "encephalopathy of prematurity" refers to encephalic gray matter abnormalities and WMA in preterm infants during the perinatal period [20]. Periventricular Leukoencephalopathy (PVL) and neuronal axonal injury are the hallmarks of this condition [21, 22].

Enlarged extracerebral space is a relatively common abnormal finding. In 2003, [23] found that very preterm infants with moderate-to-severe disability at 12 months of age (based on clinical examination) had reduced cortical and subcortical gray matter volumes and increased cerebrospinal fluid volumes compared to infants without disability or with mild disability. Enlarged extracerebral space is a relatively common abnormal finding. Anderson [24] described that in the 1998–2000 Christchurch cohort, 51% of very preterm infants had a mild enlargement of the extracerebral space, while 17% had a moderate-to-severe enlargement **Figure 2**.

MRI findings in extremely and very preterm showed that 50–80% have diffuse white matter abnormalities (WMA), which have been related to significant neurological and psychological deficits [25–27]. In preterm infants, MRI findings include diffuse and cystic white matter abnormalities, germinal matrix hemorrhage / intraventricular hemorrhage, neuronal loss, and gliosis of the gray matter (subcortical gray matter and cerebellum are the most affected). For a review visit [27].

Another characteristic of MRI in preterm babies is the volume decrease of the corpus callosum, as shown in **Figure 3**.

1.3 Katona's neurohabilitation

Katona [5] proposed the term neurohabilitation to differentiate it from rehabilitation. The main difference is that neurohabilitatory treatment should begin before the sequels of the lesion have been established, during the first 1–4 months after birth,

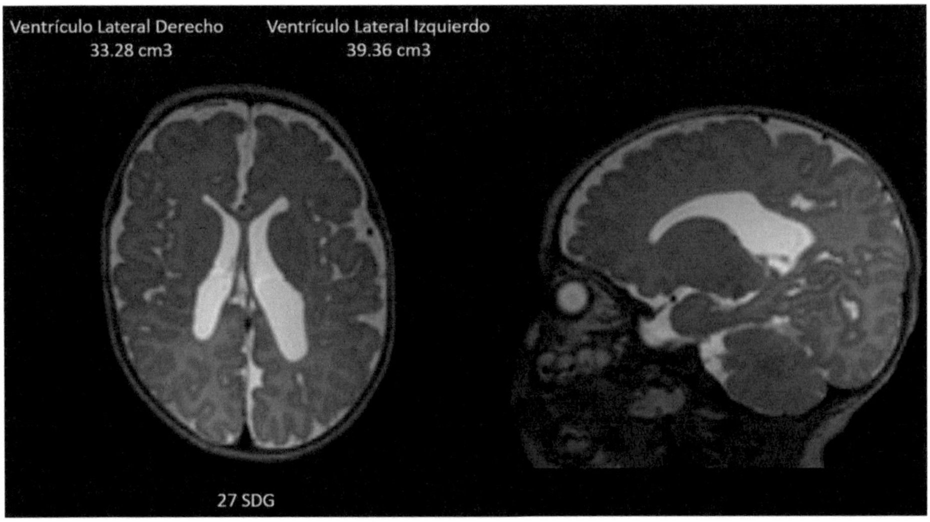

Figure 2.
Longitudinal and sagittal MRI of a preterm child of 27 weeks of gestational age. The enlargement of the lateral ventricles can be observed. The volume of the right lateral ventricle is 32.28 cm3 and 39.36 cm3 of the left lateral ventricle.

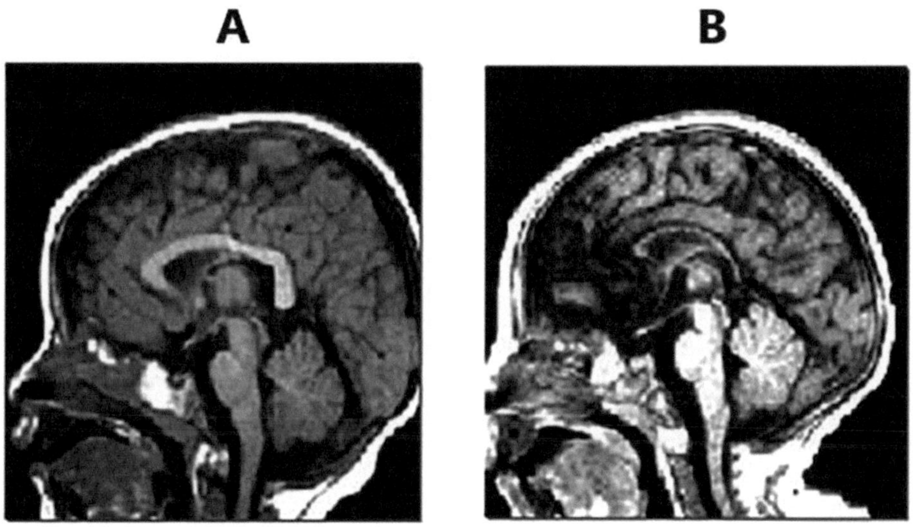

Figure 3.
Sagittal MRI of two infants at one-year-old. A corresponds to a normal child with adequate corpus callosum volume. B is the image of a preterm infant (32 weeks of gestational age) with a small corpus callosum volume.

to try to decrease or abolish the neurological sequels that perinatal brain damage may produce.

This procedure is both diagnostic and therapeutic. It evaluates muscle tone, body symmetry, attention, eye tracking, and auditory monitoring.

According to Katona [5], the therapy uses "elementary motor patterns," which are human-specific and present from 24 weeks of gestational age to 6 months. These early integrated complex movements are chains of processes in which the neck, trunk, and extremities perform complex and continual movements in certain repetitive patterns. These motor patterns have high organization, persistence, and stereotypy [28]. The developing subcortical structures control these movements. They can be activated by determined head and body positions that trigger the activation of the vestibular nuclei and their projections to the spinal cord, reticular formation, thalamus, cerebellum, and basal ganglia, whose tracts are already myelinated. Later, all these structures project into the sensorimotor cortex by myelinated axons [29]. **Figure 4** shows the neural pathways after the activation of the semicircular channels by the movements of the head.

A therapeutic program consists of training a series of neuromotor patterns each day for a certain time. Katon described 40 maneuvers to trigger the elementary motor patterns. The different positions to generate the specific neuromotor patterns are described in [30]. The repeated generation of these movements produces brain engrams that improve motor development. At the initiation of the treatment, specialized therapists conducted the Katona evaluations to obtain a diagnosis and to program 5 to 6 maneuvers that parents should learn to apply to their infants at home during the first month of therapy. After a month, the therapist evaluates the infant and selects the maneuvers for the next month, and this happens every month until the infant reaches independent walking. The therapy is intensive and specific for each infant.

Three to five maneuvers (as shown in **Figure 5**) are repeated five to six times in one therapeutic session that lasts 45 minutes and should be repeated 3 or 5 times daily. Parents learn how to perform the exercises correctly since they will treat the infant at

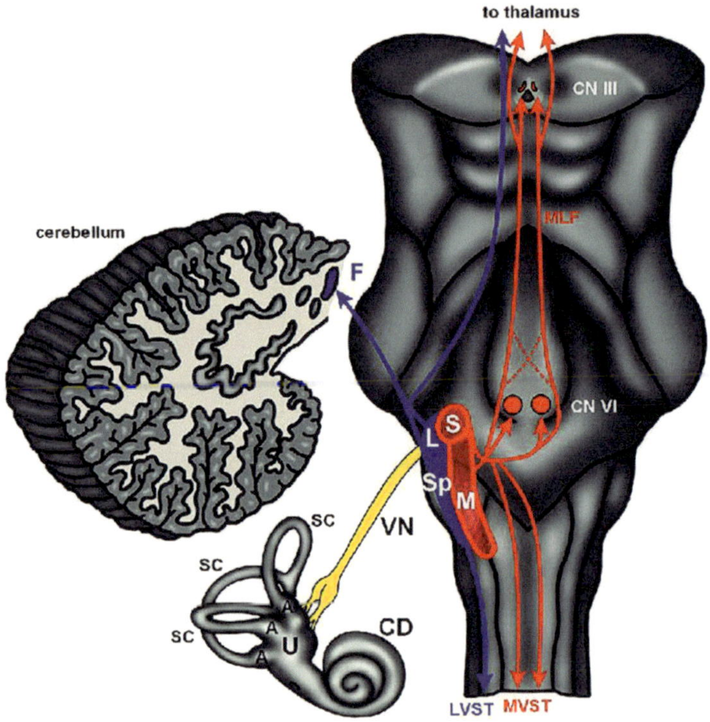

Figure 4.
Different positions of the head activate the semicircular channels (SC) that send afferent fibers by the VIII pair (Vestibular nerve, VN) to the vestibular nuclei (L, SP, S, M) in the medulla oblongata. These nuclei send descendant fibers to the spinal cord (LVST and MVST) and ascendant fibers to the nuclei of the abducens nuclei, the oculomotor nuclei, the cerebellum, and the thalamus. The Centro median thalamic nuclei send projections to the striatum and the cortex.

home. Therapy must be integrated into the infant's schedule and divided into periods according to sleeping and wakefulness patterns and feeding and nursing schedules. Each month, the infant was examined, evaluating both motor performance and visual and auditory attention and the ages at which the infant mastered various developmental milestones **Figures 5** and **6**.

2. Results

In the Neurodevelopmental Research Unit, where we work with infants, we perform multidisciplinary evaluations of the infants. The inclusion criteria are a corrected age (CA) of 2 months or less and prenatal and/or perinatal risk factors for brain damage. The exclusion criteria are genetic factors associated with brain damage, cardiovascular pathology, brain malformations, and/or chromosomal aberrations. In the first step, a pediatrician confirms these criteria. Immediately and in parallel, the multidisciplinary evaluations (pediatric, neuropediatric, psychological, electrophysiological (EEG, visual, and auditory evoked potentials), and brain MRI) and Katona's therapy begin. We follow up with infants up to 8 years old. During this period, several multidisciplinary evaluations are done. If, in those evaluations, some motor, sensory, and/ or cognitive incapacity is detected, it is immediately treated. **Figure 7** shows the different steps.

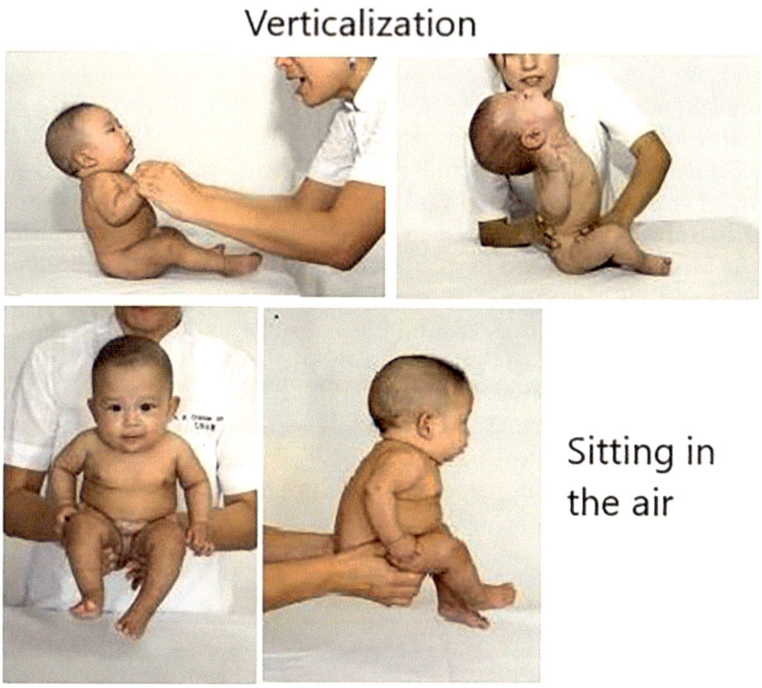

Figure 5.
Katona's positions for verticalization of the body. In the upper images are shown how the therapist should place his/her hands to activate the vertical position of the baby. The lower images show the other hand positions in the inferior extremities of the baby to obtain the "sitting in the air" position.

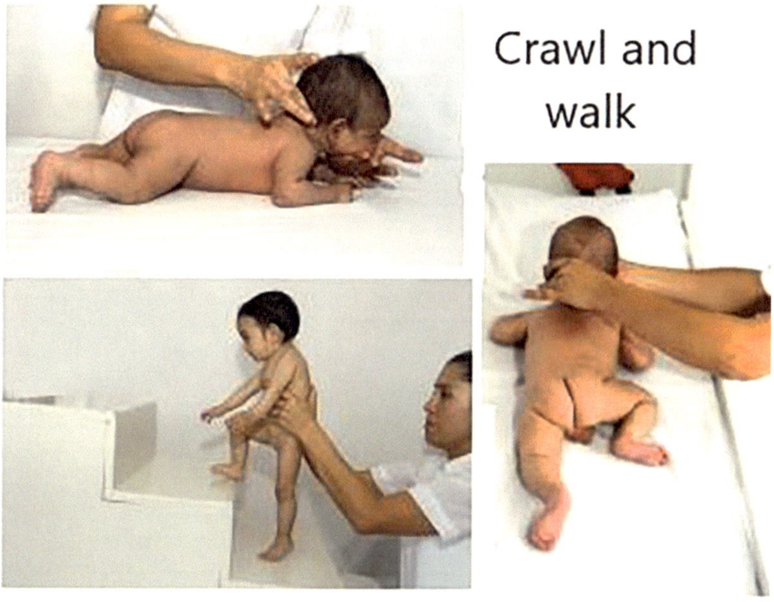

Figure 6.
Positions of the baby and hands of the therapist to improve crawling in a horizontal plane and in an ascendent ramp. It is also shown how the therapist helps the infant up a step.

The results of applying Katona's neurohabilitation have shown in several infant samples that it prevents neurological and cognitive sequels in infants with prenatal and perinatal risk factors [31–35].

Harmony [18] studied a group of 262 infants from 25 to 40 WGA with prenatal and perinatal risk factors for brain damage. In this group, the MRI showed that 80% of the subjects had some abnormal findings, particularly increased volumes of the subarachnoidal space and the lateral ventricles. Decreased volumes of the corpus callosum were also observed. Application of Katona's methodology showed that at three years old, the Mental (MDI) and Psychomotor Developmental (PDI) Indices were normal at 62% and 80%, respectively. In this sample, if those infants with slight delay were added to the normal infants, around 90% of subjects could have appropriate behavior among their peers. See **Figure 8** for these results.

In another publication related to prenatal and perinatal risk factors, where 82% of the infants had some abnormal MRI findings, we used Katona's procedure. The outcome of children at eight years old showed that 78, 76, and 78% of extremely preterm, very preterm, and late preterm, respectively, had normal neurodevelopment [36].

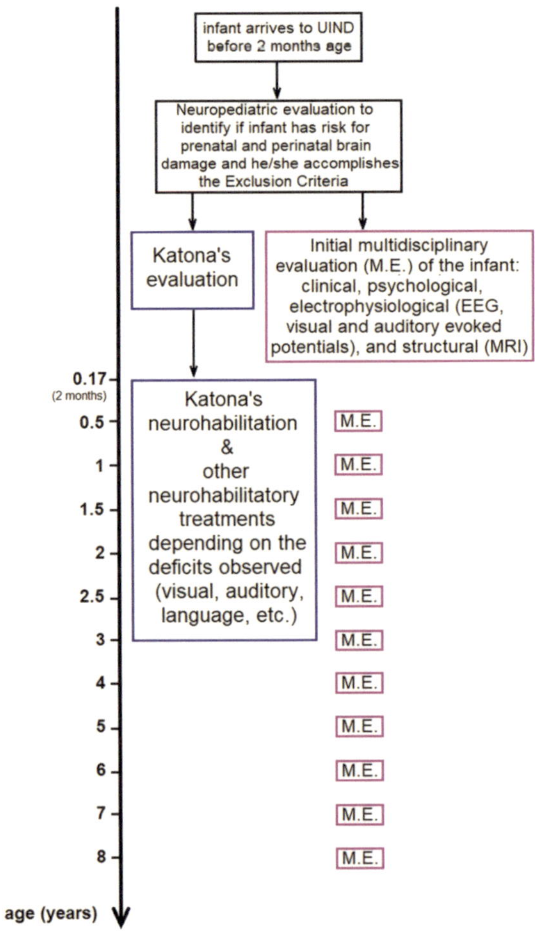

Figure 7.
This figure shows the main steps followed by the Developmental Research Unit (Unidad de Investigación en Neurodesarrollo, UIND) for the multidisciplinary evaluation and treatment of infants and their follow-up.

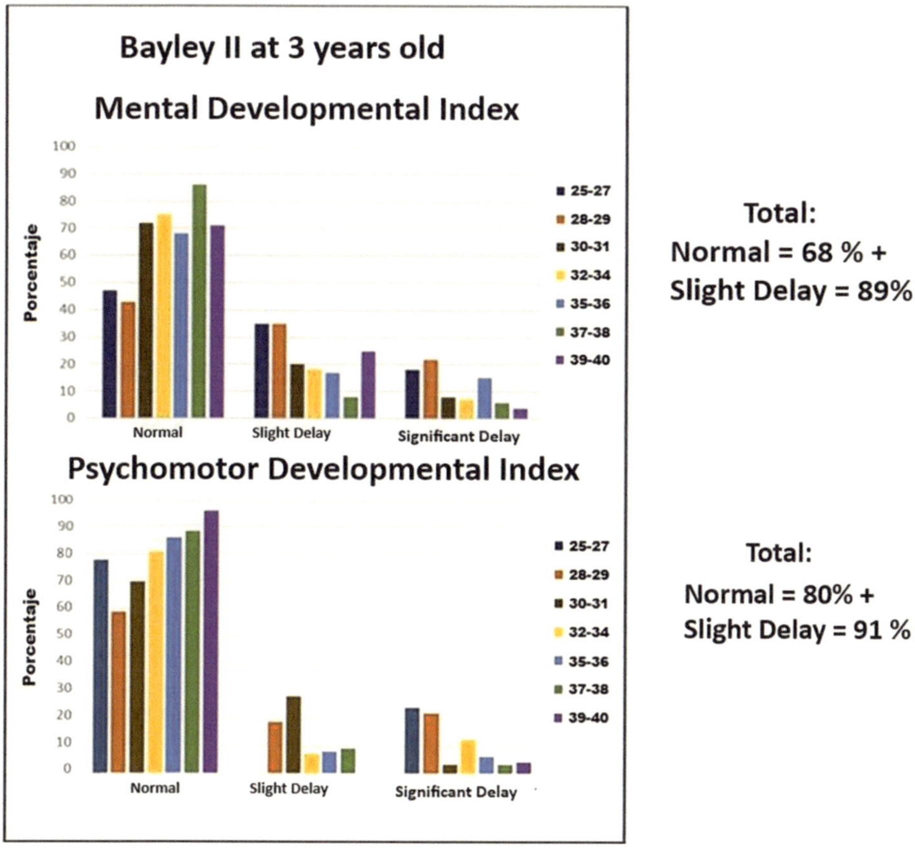

Figure 8.
Results of Bayley's II test at 3 years old of 262 preterm infants who followed Katona's therapy from 2 months to 24 months. The colors indicate the gestational age at birth in the right column. If indices of all infants (25 to 40 weeks of gestational age) were added, the total Mental Developmental Index is Normal + Accelerated = 68% + Mildly delayed 89%. The total Psychomotor Developmental Index is Normal + Accelerated = 80% + Mildly delayed 91%.

In a recent publication, we compare the outcome of 166 preterm infants with prenatal and perinatal risk factors and MRI showing structural abnormalities in 87% of the infants that were treated with Katona's procedure and a group of infants with similar brain abnormalities where parents did not approve the treatment. The parents of 128 infants accepted and received Katona's neurohabilitation treatment. The remaining 38 infants did not receive treatment. Bayley's II scales were applied in both groups at three years old. The treated infants showed normal values (100 on the MDI scale and 104 on the PDI scale), and the nontreated children were 79 on the MDI and 81 on the PDI. The differences between groups were very significant [16].

3. Discussion

The application of Katona's neurohabilitation is based on the work at home by their parents or somebody who, for at least one year, dedicated the whole day to attending the infant in care. This is necessary for the infant to receive 3 to 4 stimulation periods with the method each day. The method should continue once the infant walks independently. The exit of treatment is due to regularly administered sessions of 45 minutes several times a day. If this is not accomplished, the neurodevelopmental outcome will not be reasonable. It is important to give feedback to the parents in each evaluation. If the therapist observes that the infant is not developing reasonably, he/she should discuss the child's future with the parent engaged, which depends on adequate adhesion to the therapy.

Barrera [30] published a Spanish-language manual for this therapy, including exercise instructions. This manual has been used in our laboratory with exit.

4. Conclusions

1. Newborns with prenatal and/or perinatal risk factors have, in 80% of the cases, abnormal MRI findings suggesting brain injury.

2. Therefore, all infants with this type of risk factor should be treated immediately, as soon as possible, to decrease neurologic sequels.

3. Katona's therapy has shown to be useful in the prevention of neurological sequels in preterm babies, as well as in term infants with perinatal brain damage.

4. Katona's therapy depends on the parents' work or someone dedicated to the infant until the infant walks independently.

Acknowledgements

The author acknowledges all members of the "Unidad de Investigación en Neurodesarrollo": Catalina Alatorre-Cruz, Teresa Álvarez Vázquez, Paulina Álvarez, Alejandra Arenas, Jesús E. Barrera Reséndiz, Héctor Belmont Tamayo, Susana Castro Chavira, Enoé Cruz, Lourdes Cubero Rego, José Oliver De Leo, Laura Estrada Martínez, Thalía Fernández, Marcela García Tinoco, Claudia Calipso Gutiérrez, Saulo Hernández, Manuel Hinojosa, Eliseo Islas, Alma Janeth Moreno, María del Consuelo Pedraza, María Juana Pérez, Verónica Tonantzin Pineda, Eneida Porras Kattz, Silvia Ruiz Tovar, Elsa Ruiz.

Author details

Thalía Harmony
Unidad de Investigación en Neurodesarrollo, Departamento de Neurobiología Conductual y Cognitiva, Instituto de Neurobiología, Universidad Nacional Autónoma de México Campus Juriquilla, Querétaro, Mexico

*Address all correspondence to: thaliah@unam.mx

References

[1] Bendix I, Hadamitzky M, Herz J, et al. Adverse neuropsychiatric development following perinatal brain injury: From a preclinical perspective. Pediatric Research. 2019;**85**:198-215. DOI: 10.1038/s41390-018-0222-6nd

[2] Monroy RAE, García RJF, Valdés LA. Risk factors of brain injury in preterm infants. Archives de Investigacion Materno Infantil. 2016;**8**(3):89-95

[3] Mwaniki MK, Atieno M, Lawn JE, Newton CR. Long-term neurodevelopmental outcomes after intrauterine and neonatal insults: A systematic review. Lancet. 2012;**379**(9814):445-452. DOI: 10.1016/S0140-6736(11)61577-8. Epub 2012 Jan 13

[4] Russ JB, Ostrem BEL. Acquired brain injuries across the perinatal Spectrum: Pathophysiology and emerging therapies. Pediatric Neurology. 2023;**148**:206-214. DOI: 10.1016/j.pediatrneurol.2023.08.001

[5] Katona F. Developmental clinical neurology and neurohabilitation in the secondary prevention of pre- and perinatal injuries of brain. In: Vietze PM, Vaughan HG, editors. Early Identification of Infants with Developmental Disabilities. Philadelphia: Grune & Stratton; 1988

[6] Olusanya BO, Kancherla V, Shaheen A. Ogbo FA and Davis AC global and regional prevalence of disabilities among children and adolescents: Analysis of findings from global health databases. Frontiers in Public Health. 2022;**10**:977453. DOI: 10.3389/fpubh.2022.977453

[7] World Health Organization (WHO). The World Bank. World Report on Disability. Geneva: World Health Organization; 2011. Available from: www.who.int/disabilities/world_report/2011/report.pdf

[8] Larroque B, Ancel PY, Marret S, Marchand L, André M, Arnaud C, et al. Neurodevelopmental disabilities and special care of 5-year-old children born before 33 weeks of gestation (the EPIPAGE study): A longitudinal cohort. The Lancet. 2008;**371**:813-820. DOI: 10.1016/S0140-6736(08)60380-3

[9] Larsen ML, Wingreen R, Jensen A, et al. The effect of gestational age on major neurodevelopmental disorders in preterm infants. Pediatric Research. 2022;**91**:1906-1912. DOI: 10.1038/s41390-021-01710-4

[10] Macnab A. Pathogenesis and prevention of fetal and neonatal brain injury. In: ZamzuriIdris, editor. Advancement and New Understanding in Brain Injury. London, UK: Intech Open; 2021. DOI: 10.5772/intechopen.93840

[11] Rees P, Callan C, Chadda KR, Vaal M, Diviney J, Sabti S, et al. Preterm brain injury and neurodevelopmental outcomes: A meta-analysis. Pediatrics. 2022;**150**(6):e2022057442. DOI: 10.1542/peds.2022-057442

[12] Pressler JL. Classification of major newborn injuries. The Journal of Perinatal & Neonatal Nursing. 2008;**22**:60-67

[13] Ghajar J. Traumatic brain injury. Lancet. 2000;**356**(9233):923-929. DOI: 10.1016/S0140-6736(00)02689-1

[14] Aylward GP. Update on neurodevelopmental outcomes of infants born prematurely. Journal of

Developmental & Behavioral Pediatrics. 2014;**35**(6):392-393. DOI: 10.1097/DBP.0000000000000075

[15] Lowry RB, Bedard T, Grevers X, Crawford S, Greenway SC, Brindle ME, et al. The Alberta congenital anomalies surveillance system: A 40-year review with prevalence and trends for selected congenital anomalies, 1997-2019. Health Promotion and Chronic Disease Prevention in Canada. 2023;**43**(1):40-48. DOI: 10.24095/hpcdp.43.1.04

[16] Gonzalez-Moreira E, Harmony T, Hinojosa-Rodríguez M, Carrillo-Prado C, Juárez-Colín ME, Gutiérrez-Hernández CC, et al. Prevention of neurological sequelae in preterm infants. Brain Sciences. 2023;**13**:753. DOI: 10.3390/brainsci13050753

[17] Matsuda N, Taki A, Tsuji A, Nakajima K, Takasawa K, Morioka C, et al. Perinatal factors affecting growth and development at age 3 years in extremely low birth weight infants born small for gestational age. Clinical Pediatric Endocrinology. 2018;**27**(1):31-38. DOI: 10.1297/cpe.27.31

[18] Harmony T. Outcome of infants at risk of brain damage after Katona neurohabilitation therapy. International Journal of Neurorehabilitation. 2017;**4**:3.2017. DOI: 10.4172/2376-0281.1000277

[19] World Health Organization (WHO). Maternal Mortality, 2023. Available from: http://Maternal.mortality.(who.int)

[20] Volpe JJ. Neurology of the Newborn. 6th ed. Amsterdam, The Netherlands: Elsevier; 2018. p. 425

[21] Kinney HC, Volpe JJ. Modeling the encephalopathy of prematurity in animals: The important role of translational research. Neurology Research International. 2012;**2012**:295389. DOI: 10.1155/2012/295389

[22] Volpe JJ. The encephalopathy of prematurity--brain injury and impaired brain development inextricably intertwined. Seminars in Pediatric Neurology. 2009;**16**(4):167-178. DOI: 10.1016/j.spen.2009.09.005

[23] Inder TE, Volpe JJ, Anderson PJ. Defining the neurologic consequences of preterm birth. The New England Journal of Medicine. 2023;**389**:441-453. DOI: 10.1056/NEJMra2303347

[24] Anderson PJ. Neuropsychological outcomes of children born very preterm. Seminars in Fetal and Neonatal Medicine. 2014;**19**(2):90-96

[25] Duerden EG, Taylor MJ, Miller SP. Brain development in infants born preterm: Looking beyond injury. Seminars in Pediatric Neurology. 2013;**20**:65-74

[26] Kwon SH, Vasung L, Laura R, Ment LR, Huppi PS. The role of neuroimaging in predicting neurodevelopmental outcomes of preterm neonates. Clinics in Perinatology. 2014;**41**:257-283

[27] Hinojosa-Rodríguez M, Harmony T, Carrillo-Prado C, Darrell Van Horn J, Irimia A, Torgerson C, et al. Clinical neuroimaging in the preterm infant: Diagnosis and prognosis. Neuroimage: Clinical. 2017;**16**:355-368

[28] Porras-Kattz E, Harmony T. Neurohabilitación: un método diagnóstico y terapéutico para prevenir secuelas por lesión cerebral en el recién nacido y el lactante. Boletín Médico del Hospital Infantil de México. 2007;**64**:44-54

[29] Kirsch V, Keeser D, Hergenroeder T, Erat D, Ertl-Wagner B, Brandt T, et al.

Structural and functional connectivity mapping of the vestibular circuitry from human brainstem to cortex. Brain Structure & Function. 2015;**5**:3-16. DOI: 10.1007/s00429-014-0971-x

[30] Barrera JE. Terapia Neurohabilitatoria. México: UNAM; 2010

[31] Pérez-Martínez JA, Zanabria-Salcedo MA. Sistema de diagnóstico y tratamiento del desarrollo temprano de Ferenc Katona. Plastic & Rest Neuroplasticity. 2004;**3**(1 y 2):59-62

[32] Alvarado-Ruiz GA, Martínez-Vázquez I, Sánchez C, Solís-Chan M, Mandujano Valdés M. The complex elementary human movements. Normal postnatal development. Preliminary report of nine Mexican infants. Salud Ment. 2012;**35**(2):99-107

[33] Karmel B, Gardner JM. Neurobehavioral assessment in the neonatal period- the impact of Ferenc Katona. Ideggyógyászati Szemle. 2005;**23**:315

[34] Acosta González CE. Intervención por el método Katona en bebés prematuros con factores de riesgo de daño neurológico. Tesis Universidad de Guadalajara. 2022. Available from: https://hdl.handle.net/20.500.12104/90939

[35] Harmony T, Barrera-Reséndiz J, Juárez-Colín ME, Carrillo-Prado C, Pedraza-Aguilar MC, Asprón Ramírez A, et al. Longitudinal study of children with perinatal brain damage in whom early neurohabilitation was applied: Preliminary report. Neuroscience Letters. 2016;**611**:59-67. DOI: 10.1016/j.neulet.2015.11.013

[36] Harmony T. Early diagnosis and treatment of infants with prenatal and perinatal risk factors for brain damage at the neurodevelopmental research unit in Mexico. NeuroImage. 2021;**135**:17984. DOI: 10.1016/j.neuroimage.2021.117984